111 Dumbbell Workouts

For the Shy Gym Girl

Your Strength Training Guide to Build Muscle, Burn Fat and Grow Confidence.

By Sophie Smith

DISCLAIMER

The information in this book is not intended to diagnose or treat any medical conditions. Always seek the advice of a medical professional before making drastic lifestyle changes. The author of this book accepts no liability for injury.

Before You Start!

Before you jump into your workouts, I'd like to give you a present!

I believe that a peaceful mind is just as important as a strong body, so I want to gift you a guided meditation to help you get back into alignment whenever you feel yourself slipping.

It's less than 10 minutes long and I want you to have it because I know how disheartening it can be to feel like you've stopped making progress.

This alignment meditation will give you the chance to reset and get right back on track whenever you listen to it.

Just email the word 'Alignment' to sophie@strongandstretchy.co.uk to receive this gift!

Join our Community!

It can be isolating and daunting getting into the gym and fitness in general by yourself, so I'd like to invite you to join a community of women who support and motivate each other online (and hopefully one day in person!).

Just email 'Community' to sophie@strongandstretchy.co.uk and I'll add you into the free Facebook group!

I can't wait for you to join our supportive family!

X

QR Codes!

Throughout this book you'll find many QR codes, a code for each movement in fact! When you scan a QR code using the camera on your mobile phone, you will be able to watch a video of the movement being performed.

I've always found that a visual demonstration is the easiest way to understand a movement so I hope you find this feature useful.

If you don't have a camera phone don't worry, there's step by step instructions to help you learn each movement!

<u>Here's a QR code to help you practice viewing the videos:</u>

Step 1) Open up the camera app on your phone.

Step 2) Hold your phone up to this QR code to scan it so that you can see the code on your screen. You'll see a small pop up saying 'Youtube' on your screen, click on that to watch the video!

Contents

Introduction

Wandering around the gym with major anxiety because you have no idea where to start. Desperately wanting to make positive changes in your body but you're just not sure how. Sound familiar?

You're not alone. In fact, according to an Independent study, one in four women avoid exercising due to the fear of being judged. One in four!! That's a whole lot of women who will neglect their amazing body due to lack of confidence. But by learning how to move your body effectively, your confidence can truly sky rocket!

The good news is that working out in the gym doesn't need to be complicated to be effective, and I'm certainly not here to tell you to 'just suck it up' and throw yourself into the main weights room and figure it all out. I've been that shy gym girl who couldn't think of anything worse than sweating it out in front of all the 'gym bros' when I really had no idea how to perform certain exercises or use the gym equipment. And whilst I promise you that no one is actually watching what you're doing in the gym (we're all too self focussed for that!), by starting simple, with minimal equipment in a space that you feel comfortable in, you can gradually adapt to the gym life and gain confidence. You'll do this by becoming familiar with more movements and through seeing positive changes in your body.

When I first started my gym journey I spent years doing random exercises for little benefit because I didn't know what I was doing and I had no confidence to ask for help. I want to change that story for you, by starting you off how I wish I had, with simple, yet effective strength training sessions.

In this book you'll find a variety of workouts that you can do in the corner of the gym until you feel more confident moving into the main weights room (which, by the way, won't seem half as scary as it might do now once you've got yourself into a good training routine!).

All you've gotta do is grab some dumbbells and a bench and find yourself a space that you feel comfortable in. If you don't have access to a gym bench you can use the floor or a different stable surface for a couple of the movements where 'bench' is written.

How to use this book

*Although the main purpose of this book is to provide you with 111 dumbbell workouts, I wanted to make sure that you have the basic knowledge needed to make your training effective, so you'll also find some information on nutrition, making training programmes, how often you'll need to workout to hit your goals and more. If you're only here for **the workouts** you might not feel like reading through all of the other information, in which case you can flick straight to **page 33** and start your sessions right away! If you would like to learn the strength training basics that can help you to build muscle, burn fat and grow confidence in the gym, just keep reading!*

*I've included video demonstrations of each listed movement in the **Movement Glossary**, which starts on **page 73**, rather than illustrations because I know how frustrating it can be to not understand a movement and I always find that videos are the most useful - just scan the QR code under the movement to watch a demonstration! When you scan the code to watch the video you'll also be able to see an explanation of the muscles that the movement uses in the video description. If you'd like to quickly find the page of a certain movement just flick to the **Glossary** on **page 99** to find the page number!*

Life is too short to avoid moving your body because you're not sure how to. You deserve to feel strong, sexy and powerful by realizing just how much your body can do. This book will give you the guidance you need to do just that.

So get your workout playlist ready, put on a training outfit that makes you feel cute, and get ready to really transform your body (*oh, and don't forget your headphones!!!*)

Part One
The Strength Training Basics

Part One
Chapter One

Rocket Fuel

You are a rocket.

Smoking hot, full of energy and seriously impressive to look at. And if you don't feel that way about yourself yet, maybe you're just not giving yourself enough fuel.

Fuel for a strength training journey comes in many forms but in this chapter we'll be focussing on just two, because these are really the most important.

The first form is the energy you give yourself through your words. And I don't even mean spoken words, but the way you talk to yourself in your head.

So often, we tell ourselves that we aren't capable of something before we've physically proven that's the case. We talk down to ourselves in a way that we'd never talk to our friends or family and beat ourselves up for not being perfect or for looking a certain way.

But I'm here to tell you that that lack of self appreciation will lower your vibration and hinder your progress in the gym.

Why? Because if you're working out because you hate your body, you'll constantly be chasing a new ideal that you'll simply never reach (because there will always be a new ideal to chase!). You likely won't be able to enjoy the process of working out because you'll be constantly chasing this end goal and will lack motivation and energy to train if you're so focussed on the things that you *don't* see in yourself.

But do you know what *does* boost your energy and make working out dare I say it.. fun? Telling yourself that *you've got this.* That you **are** capable and strong and attractive. Because YOU ARE.

Complimenting yourself for showing up, for not giving up on the days that you don't feel like moving, or for pushing through one last rep of a movement that is really challenging you, is a great way to build your self appreciation and your relationship with the gym!

Everyone starts somewhere, and no matter how inexperienced or un confident you feel right now, with some dedication, consistency and a simple plan, you can become your best self in no time. You just have to make the choice to start. And you're here, so well done for taking that step!

From this point on I challenge you to talk to yourself how you'd talk to your best friend, or to your mom, dad or child. Would you tell them they're useless if they didn't get something right the first time? Or that they'll never be in great shape? Or that they don't deserve to take the time to fit a workout in?

No, you wouldn't (I hope!), so from now on your task is to not talk to yourself like that either!

It's all about self love over here. And I don't mean the superficial only-for-the-gram self love. It's about forming real, deep love and respect for yourself. And you'll do that by consistently showing up for and talking nicely to yourself.

There will be days that you feel like giving up on your strength training journey and I'm not telling you for one second that you need to pretend to be overly positive on those days. Accept them as an inevitable part of your journey, but show yourself that you respect yourself enough to keep moving forward, even if you have to take breaks.

When you're months or years down the line you will look back on the times you pushed through with so much admiration for yourself that your self love will be through the roof!

The best part? When you're in love with yourself and have a load of self respect and admiration, you will attract other things and people that love and appreciate you too ~ But that's a whole other story for a whole other book!

In short, you are worthy of the time to work on yourself. You are deserving of the body of your dreams. And you can have it all! Promise me, and promise yourself, that from this point on, you will start fueling your mind with positive energy through kind self-talk. Your body is a blessing and so is the ability to move! I can't wait for you to truly realize that if you don't already, because it really is the most fulfilling realization in the world.

Use the lines below to write a promise to yourself now, that you will feed yourself with kind words, even if only in your head, and that this will be the start of fueling your journey the right way!

Here's an example:

From this date on, I promise myself that I will be dedicated to becoming the best version of myself. I will be kind to myself and I won't give up on myself because I deserve to feel happy and strong and sexy.

Now write yours here:

_____

_____

_____

Signed:..   Date:...

You can reflect back on this promise anytime you feel like giving up. One thing I can guarantee you, is that you will feel so incredibly proud when you've reached your fitness goals and you look back at this. You will be full of self appreciation for seeing your goals through and keeping your word to yourself.

So that's the first type of fuel you will now be using - positive energy and kind words. Now let's discuss another type, something more physical!

Food!

Something that took me a long time to figure out is the importance of a good diet when looking to achieve my dream physique. And when I say a 'good diet', I don't mean eating salad all day everyday whilst sniffing sweet treats to try and satisfy your sugar cravings. From experience I can tell you that will only end in a miserable binge and probably a lot of crying.

A 'good' diet to me means consuming enough nutrients and energy to perform your workouts without feeling fatigued and grouchy, and your diet really doesn't have to be restrictive to achieve this. The 80/20 rule is a great place to start - this means eating 80% nutritious food and 20% treats! This will mean that if you want chocolate after dinner one day, or pizza with a friend, or ice cream at the movies, or whatever else makes your soul happy, you can eat your heart out and get right back on track with your next meal. It can really help with getting rid of any guilt that comes with eating 'unhealthy' foods and by not consistently restricting yourself, you're limiting the urge to binge eat!

The actual amount of food you'll need to consume to fuel your body will depend on different factors but before you work out how much you'll need, you'll have to get clear on your main goal. Have a read through the options below and decide on this first!

Weight loss

If your main goal is to lose weight, you'll need to be in a **calorie deficit**, which means consuming less calories than you burn throughout the day (in your workouts or otherwise). You can calculate the amount of calories you'll need to consume to be in a calorie deficit using a lot of online calculators, like this one at FitWatch - https://www.fitwatch.com/calculator/calorie-deficit or my personal favorite, this one at Legion Athletics - https://legionathletics.com/tools/calorie-calculator/. Or if you don't hate math and want to learn the calculation process yourself, jump to Page 94 to read the full explanation.

A lot of studies show that eating up to 500 calories less than the calories needed to maintain your weight is a suitable suggested deficit. Though I'm not a qualified nutritionist so can't provide advice on this as such, I would always suggest using a percentage deficit rather than a set amount because we are all different and have different factors to take into account. You want to make sure you're consuming enough calories to continue fueling yourself to stay healthy and if you already don't weigh very much or burn very many calories, 500 less calories could be a huge amount.

Founder of Built Lean, Marc Perry also suggests going into a calorie deficit *percentage* range of 20%-35% fewer calories than your total calorie burn if you want to lose weight healthily. The above calculators can help you to work out what your daily calorie burn is so that you can calculate your deficit percentage, or you can skip to page 94 to work it out for yourself!

The aim is to gradually make positive changes to your body and lifestyle and the last thing you want to do is starve yourself. Remember it's all about self love over here - be patient and work *with* your body as you make your desired changes.

Weight Gain

If your goal is weight gain, you'll need to be in a **calorie surplus**, which means consuming more calories than you burn throughout the day. You can use the

Legion Athletics calculator - https://legionathletics.com/tools/calorie-calculator/, or the explanation on page 94 to work out how many calories you'll need to consume to achieve this!

Building Muscle and Burning Fat

If your goal is to build muscle **and** lose fat to achieve a toned or curvier look, you have two main options.

Option 1) Go through 'bulk and cut' phases.

This is where you eat in a big surplus (consuming more calories than your body burns), which will result in faster weight gain, which, if eating sufficient protein, should lead to more muscle growth in a shorter period of time compared to if you weren't eating in a surplus, but it will also make you gain some fat.

Once you've 'bulked' you would then go through a 'cutting' phase, where your protein intake remains high to limit muscle loss but your body fat drops, leaving behind your curves (muscles) in all the right places.

Though this is perhaps the most common option for bikini competing athletes, I personally don't feel this is the best way to go if you're just starting out in your strength training journey. Changing your body so much over these time periods often leads to body image issues and you could feel very restricted when 'cutting'. And we don't like restriction over here, this is all about creating a lifestyle. This is just my preference though and of course you may end up loving this option if you try it!

Option 2) Lean bulk.

This means gradually building your muscle without gaining too much fat as you work towards your dream physique by still eating in a surplus, but a much smaller one compared to if you were bulking. This is the option I personally prefer as I feel it's more sustainable as a lifestyle compared to bulking/cutting and I also feel it's more beginner friendly. It may take a little longer to see results but over time you'll achieve the physique you want without dreading the different phases of your training cycle.

A good place to start if you're looking to gradually build muscle without gaining too much fat, would be to consume an extra 10% of your daily Total Estimated Energy Expenditure (TDEE) as well as between 0.8-1.2g of protein per pound of bodyweight.

To work out your TDEE and how many calories you'll need to eat to achieve a slower muscle build and fat burn, visit https://legionathletics.com/tools/calorie-calculator/ and select the 'slow' option - or jump to page 94 if you'd like to work it out yourself!

Pizza is encouraged over here!

As previously mentioned, restriction isn't what you should aim for no matter your fitness goal! And something that will be super important in your strength training journey is making sure you're consuming enough carbohydrates and protein to give yourself enough energy to workout. Even if your goal is to lose weight, carbs are still encouraged and in fact *needed* to give you enough fuel to train! I see so many people (my old self included), avoiding carbs and undereating with the aim of losing weight, but this will very likely end in misery and binging. Food really is your friend, with carbs being your main source of energy and protein being the building blocks for your muscles - don't neglect it!

Speaking of protein, this is really important when strength training, as you'll need to consume enough for your muscles to grow and repair.

A good general guideline for a strength trainer looking to gradually build muscle would be to consume between *0.8 - 1.2 grams of protein per pound of bodyweight*. So if you weigh 145 lbs, you would want to consume between 116-174 grams of protein per day, with the majority of the rest of your diet consisting of high quality carbohydrates to give you sufficient energy (around 40-60%), and the rest of your food being healthy fats (around 20-30%). Of course there are micronutrients and other factors to be considered when it comes to your diet, but to keep this book simple we will just focus on the basics.

Everyone's body responds differently to protein and different nutrients so as long as you're hitting the minimum recommended amount, you can make small adjustments once you get used to how much your body needs.

Calculate your daily protein intake here:

Pick a number between 0.8 and 1.2 X *your bodyweight in lbs* = *Your daily protein target.*

Summary

So you've hopefully worked out how many calories and how much protein you'll need to eat each day to hit your fitness goals, well done!

Although nutrition can seem complicated, it really doesn't need to be. Try to hit your calorie targets and eat enough protein but don't let your diet rule your life. If you're not competing for a bodybuilding bikini competition you really don't need to be completely strict all the time. I'm a huge foodie and I've found that I enjoy working out the most when I actually allow myself treats when I want them.

If you ever overeat, just get back on track the next meal or the next day, don't restrict or punish yourself! Life is too short to not eat cake and pizza - just enjoy all foods in moderation!

Finally, remember that how you talk to yourself will also have a huge impact on your strength training journey. You can reflect back on the promise you made yourself earlier in this chapter if you're ever feeling unmotivated!

Part One
Chapter Two

Your Workout Schedule

"Failing to prepare is preparing to fail" - Benjamin Franklin

It pains me to think of the hundreds, probably thousands of hours that I've spent exercising in my life without any intention behind my workouts. Meaning yes, I've been burning some calories, maybe building a teeny tiny bit of muscle here and there, but overall making minimal progress. And whilst movement is never a waste, why spend your time aimlessly working out to see little effect, when you could spend your energy on a planned workout that you know can bring you great results?

You're spending the same amount of time working out whether you're doing it right or wrong anyway (if not less time when doing it right!), so you may as well make it worth it, right?

That's where programming comes in. Programming is simply creating a workout plan that aligns with your goals. And it doesn't need to be complicated.

I've tried many programs, from working out twice a day whilst on a leaf diet (which every time resulted in burnout and a lot of crying), to two hour long workouts that left me dreading the gym beforehand everytime (and often skipping the workout), to great plans where I've seen real progress.

The key with planning your strength training sessions is to make them fit into your lifestyle, not the other way around! If you know you get bored doing something after 45 minutes, plan in 45 minute gym sessions so that you can stay motivated and actually enjoy training! Or if you know that you're more motivated in the mornings, slot your sessions in then! Work *with* yourself and your life to add in your training sessions so that they can become part of your lifestyle.

When it comes to planning your training schedule, there are two types of training options that I've seen so many people make progress with when strength training.
These options are:

1) **Body Part Split** - This training style is when you target certain body parts in each session. It allows you to train on consistent days as you can rest the body parts that were targeted in the previous workout. For example you could have 3 lower body days and two upper body days in the pattern of lower, upper, lower, upper, lower.

2) **Full Body Workouts** - This training style is when you do a full body workout each session, your workouts may be a little longer but could be a great option if you want to train on less days each week and still ensure you're targeting as many muscles as possible.

The secret to success behind whatever style of program you pick, is to keep it **consistent.**

But before you choose what style of training schedule you'd like to try, you might be wondering *'well how often do I need to workout to achieve my goals?'* The annoying answer to that question is that there really is no one size fits all because it depends on what your goals are, as well as factors like how active you are outside of the gym, how much rest you get, what you eat etc..

A good goal would be to workout between 3-5 times per week. This is because according to a Sports Medicine study, the "current body of evidence indicates that frequencies of training twice a week promote superior hypertrophic outcomes to once a week." So basically, strength training more than once a week means more muscle growth, which I know seems super obvious, but nevertheless it suggests that **each muscle group should be targeted at least twice per week in order to grow.** Therefore if you schedule in at least 3 sessions per week, you're giving yourself the best chance of targeting the muscles that you want to grow, which is great if your goal is to build muscle or appear more toned. For example if you want to build a booty, you'll need to schedule in at least two glute focussed movements each week (as well as eating enough calories and protein, allowing sufficient rest etc..) At least three effective sessions will also give you the chance to burn a good amount of calories throughout the week, which is great if your goal is fat loss or just generally staying fit.

So the first step in creating your plan is deciding how many days per week you can commit to. It's always best to start off with less, rather than to schedule in six or seven sessions, for you to stick to the plan for a few weeks before realizing it's unrealistic and too tiring and giving up. Rest is also extremely important so try to schedule your sessions at least 24-48 hours apart to allow for recovery.

You can write how many training sessions you want to commit to each week here:

Progressive Overload

Another vital factor for muscle growth and general fitness progression is progressive overload. This means adding more reps, heavier weight, less rest time, more intensity, or another form of extra resistance or intensity into your training, to ensure that you're regularly, progressively challenging your muscles.

Without progressive overload you won't be making the progress you desire as your muscles will become used to the resistance and won't grow as quickly as you want them to.

A good general marker for when to progressively overload a movement is when you can repeat 12 repetitions of the movement with relative ease and good form. For example, if you can perform 4 sets of 12 reps of bicep curls without feeling overly challenged or really struggling on the last few reps, it's time to add more weight and drop the reps back down to between 8-10. Then build the reps back up with that new weight and repeat the process. It's not always about pushing to failure (when you can't perform the last rep of a movement), but the last few reps of each set you do should be a struggle.

You don't need to attempt huge advancements every session, but even small amounts of progressive overload consistently, will lead to huge changes over time! So even if you're just adding in an extra rep on each set, or a small amount of weight to your movements, you can make a lot of progress!

Reps and Sets

So how many times should you repeat each exercise to ensure progression?

To build muscle size (hypertrophy) it is recommended that you perform 8-12 repetitions of each exercise for 3-5 sets with a 1-2 minute break in between sets. This is a good guideline to work off for any strength training session.
If you're training for strength and power you would want to lower the reps and increase the rest time in between sets.

The workouts in this book have been written with mostly 8-10 repetitions and 3-4 sets - this is a general guideline and you can tailor this based on how you feel with each movement.

Rest

Rest is actually just as important as movement when it comes to strength training, because it's when our body repairs and the muscles grow.
According to Bodybuilding.com, the most effective rest period for increasing power and strength is between 2 to 5 minutes between sets, and between 30 to 90 seconds between sets for muscle growth.

The workouts in this book can help with strength, power, muscle growth, fat burning and more, so you'll want to pick a suitable rest time in between your exercises depending on your goals.

Something that has been programmed for me by highly experienced weightlifting coaches is 2-3 minutes rest for my bigger lifts (like squats, deadlifts, hip thrusts and chest press), and between 1-2 minutes rest for my accessory movements. This complies with Bodybuilding.com's recommendations and it's always worked well for me so that could be a good place for you to start. We're all different so have a go and see what works for you!

Structure

Once you've determined how frequently you're able to workout, it's time to plan your sessions. Of course my hope is that you use the workouts provided in the next chapter of this book to make up your plan, but I'd also love you to be able to plan your own, as I'm sure you'll want to mix things up at some point! You can use the exercises from the Movement Glossary (page 73) to plan your own sessions when you're ready!

A good general structure for a strength training workout is:

A 5-10 minute warm up:

This should start with a **pulse/temperature raising activity** like star jumps, gentle jogging, skipping or rowing for around 5 minutes. These examples of activities are good to use as they're **aerobic movements** and will help to get the muscles warm.

Some gentle **dynamic stretches** should then be included to increase joint and muscle mobility.

Muscle activation should then be included, for example if you're wanting to build a booty, activating the glutes is necessary before performing your actual glute building lifts. Activating them will help with mind-muscle connection when you're performing the movements in the workout and will make it easier to build the muscles up as they'll be recruited when performing the lift.

Then finish your warmup with some **potentiation**. This means performing a movement that you'll be doing in your main workout, in your warm up, but with no weight, then building up the weight until you reach the weight you'll be performing your main sets with. For example, if you had dumbbell front squats in your main workout, you could perform some bodyweight front squats, then some front squats with lighter dumbbells before using the weight you'll need for your main sets.

Mimicking the movement pattern of your main lift as you warm up will get your body familiar with it and will get you accustomed to the weight as it increases so that your body is prepared and you can perform your main lifts effectively.

One or two main compound movements:
Squats, Deadlifts and Chest Press are often referred to as the 'big three' lifts in weightlifting so it's great to always include one of these, or a variation of them in each session. I will personally always make sure I'm squatting, deadlifting or hip thrusting in every workout, even if it's a variety of those lifts, like Dumbbell Thrusters instead of Back Squats or Romanian Deadlifts instead of a standard Deadlift.

These movements are great all rounders that help you to build a strong core as well as a strong back, legs, glutes and more and in my opinion, should always be the foundation of a good strength training workout.

Accessorize:
Then add 2-4 accessory movements targeting the same or different muscle groups than those that were targeted in your main compound movement. The purpose of adding accessory movements is to add variety to the workout and overload the muscles that you're targeting for growth.

Cool Down:

A cool down is super important for returning your body back to its normal state after training. Take 5-10 minutes at the end of each session to do some gentle movement that lowers your heart rate and prepares your body for the rest of the day to prevent injury. Bonus points if you fit in some stretching to work on your flexibility too!

There are of course other ways to plan a strength training session but this is an example of how to plan a simple, yet very effective one!

Examples of Standard Dumbbell Strength Training Workouts:
(All of the below exercises can be found in the Movement Glossary on page 73, with step by step instructions on how to perform them as well as a video demonstration).

If you prefer a **body part split plan** where you have set leg days, upper body days etc, a typical glute day workout could look something like this:

Warmup
4x8-12 Dumbbell Back Squats
3x8-12 Dumbbell Hip Thrusts
3x8-12 Single Leg Dumbbell Hip Thrust
3x8-12 Standing Dumbbell Lateral Hip Abduction
3x 30 second Wall Sit
Cooldown

Or if you prefer a **full body plan** where each workout is a full body session, a typical workout could look something like this:

Warmup
4x8-12 Back Squats
3x8-12 Dumbbell Hip Thrusts
3x8-12 Single Leg Dumbbell Hip Thrusts
3x8-12 Dumbbell Bent Over Rows
3x8-12 Dumbbell Chest Press
3x30 each side Russian Twists
Cooldown

Here is an example of a beginners _full body_ dumbbell strength training weekly plan:

Full Body	REST	Full Body	REST	REST	Full Body	Rest

Mon	Tues	Wed	Thurs	Fri	Sat	Sun
Warm Up	REST	Warm Up	REST	REST	Warm Up	REST
Dumbbell Back Squats	REST	Dumbbell Hip Thrusts	REST	REST	Barbell Romanian Deadlifts	REST
Dumbbell Thrusters	REST	Dumbbell Romanian Deadlifts	REST	REST	Dumbbell Hip Thrusts	REST
Dumbbell Bent Over Rows	REST	Single Leg Dumbbell Romanian Deadlift	REST	REST	Single Leg Dumbbell Hip Thrusts	REST
Dumbbell Chest Press	REST	Dumbbell Shoulder Press	REST	REST	Dumbbell Bent Over Rows	REST
Dumbbell Reverse Flys	REST	Dumbbell Chest Press	REST	REST	Dumbbell Shoulder Press	REST
Russian Twists	REST	Lying Leg Raises	REST	REST	Single Arm Dumbbell Bent Over Rows	REST
Cool Down/Stretch	REST	Cool Down/Stretch	REST	REST	Cool Down/Stretch	REST

Here is an example of a split body part dumbbell strength training weekly plan:

Legs and shoulders	Glutes and Back	Rest	Upper Body	Glutes	Rest	Rest

Mon	Tues	Wed	Thurs	Fri	Sat	Sun
Warm Up	Warm Up	REST	Warm Up	Warm Up	REST	REST
Dumbbell Back Squats	Dumbbell Romanian Deadlifts	REST	Dumbbell Thrusters	Dumbbell Romanian Deadlifts	REST	REST
Reverse Lunges	Rear Foot Elevated Bulgarian Split Squats	REST	Dumbbell Chest Press	Dumbbell Hip Thrusts	REST	REST
Dumbbell Shoulder Press	Dumbbell Bent Over Row	REST	Dumbbell Bent Over Row	Rear Foot Elevated Bulgarian Split Squats	REST	REST
Dumbbell Lateral Shoulder Raise	Dumbbell Chest Press	REST	Single Arm Dumbbell Bent Over Row	Clam Shells	REST	REST
Dumbbell Thrusters	Dumbbell Reverse Fly	REST	Lying Leg Raises	Russian Twists	REST	REST
Cool Down/Stretch	Cool Down/Stretch	REST	Cool Down/Stretch	Cool Down/Stretch	REST	REST

Summary

- These plans are generic examples of what a typical week could look like for a beginner/intermediate strength trainer looking to build muscle and/or lose fat with either a split body or full body programme using dumbbells. The training days and exercises used can vary based on your preference and schedule etc..

- Rest is just as important as the workout! Allow at least 24 hours between sessions but ideally at least 48 hours before training the same muscle group.

- Each muscle needs to be resistance trained at least twice per week to ensure hypertrophy (growth).

- Between 3-5 sessions per week can allow for weight loss, muscle growth or both. Start with less and build up once working out becomes part of your lifestyle.

- Progressive overload is key. You must ensure you're adding it each week to continue making progress.

Flip the page to make your own workout schedule!

Top tip: Make your plan realistic, even if it seems a little unambitious. It's much more sustainable and effective to schedule in three high quality training sessions per week than to schedule in five or six and go all out for two weeks, before getting burned out and concluding that strength training just isn't for you! Remember the aim is to fit training around your lifestyle, not the other way around! If you find you can easily stick to three sessions, you can always add more!

Create Your Own Workout Schedule!

Now it's time for you to create your workout schedule. To receive a print out that allows you to schedule the whole 12 weeks, please email sophie@strongandstretchy.co.uk.
You can use the following pages to plan your first four weeks if you're reading this book in the print version!

If you're not yet confident enough to plan your own workouts together, not to worry! In the next chapter you'll find 111 workouts that you can use to create your plan. All you need to do then is show up and perform the movements, working out suitable weights for each exercise as you learn!

Monday	Tuesday	Wednesday	Thursday	Friday	Saturday	Sunday

Monday	Tuesday	Wednesday	Thursday	Friday	Saturday	Sunday

Monday	Tuesday	Wednesday	Thursday	Friday	Saturday	Sunday

Monday	Tuesday	Wednesday	Thursday	Friday	Saturday	Sunday

Part Two
111 Workouts

111 Workouts

I know how daunting it can be trying to get into a good strength training routine when you feel overwhelmed by all of the different gym equipment. But you can make really great progress with minimal equipment until you feel ready to move into other areas in the gym!

For all of the workouts in this chapter all you need is a pair of dumbbells (and a good music playlist of course!).

A couple of the exercises listed would be best performed on a gym bench or plyometric box but alternatively can be performed on the gym floor or on another stable surface.

If you're unsure on how to do any of the movements listed, just flick to the movement glossary on page 73 to read step by instructions and watch a video demonstration!

Remember to do a warm up before each session and a cool down after, and allow sufficient rest time in between each exercise.

Find a space that you feel comfortable in, grab your dumbbells, and let's get moving!

For full body workouts visit page 34

For glute focussed workouts visit page 56

For lower body focussed workouts visit page 61

For upper body focussed workouts visit page 66

Full Body Workouts

Workout 1)

4x10 Sumo Squats (2-3 minute rest between sets)
3x10 Dumbbell Romanian Deadlifts (1-2 minute rest between sets)
3x10 each side Bulgarian Split Squat (1-2 minute rest between sets)
3x10 Dumbbell Shoulder Press (1-2 minute rest between sets)
3x10 Lateral Shoulder Raises (1-2 minute rest between sets)
3x30 Russian Twists (1-2 minute rest between sets)

Workout 2)

4x10 Dumbbell Romanian Deadlift (2-3 minute rest between sets)
3x10 each side Single Leg Dumbbell Romanian Deadlift (1-2 minute rest between sets)
3x10 each side Standing Hip Abduction (1-2 minute rest between sets)
3x10 Dumbbell Bent Over Row (1-2 minute rest between sets)
3x10 each side Dumbbell Single Arm Bent Over Row (1-2 minute rest between sets)
3x30 Russian Twists (1-2 minute rest between sets)

Workout 3)

4x10 Sumo Squats (2-3 minute rest between sets)
3x10 Dumbbell Romanian Deadlifts (1-2 minute rest between sets)
3x10 each side Bulgarian Split Squat (1-2 minute rest between sets)
3x10 Dumbbell Bent Over Row (1-2 minute rest between sets)
3x10 Bent Over Rear Fly (1-2 minute rest between sets)
3x10 Lying Leg Raise (1-2 minute rest between sets)

Workout 4)

4x10 3-1 tempo Sumo Squats (lower into the movement for 3 seconds then stand up in 1) (2-3 minute rest between sets)
3x10 Single Leg Dumbbell Hip Thrust (1-2 minute rest between sets)
(replace with single leg glute bridges if you don't want to use a bench!)
3x10 each side Standing Hip Abduction (1-2 minute rest between sets)
3x10 Dumbbell Shoulder Press (1-2 minute rest between sets)
3x10 Lateral Shoulder Raises (1-2 minute rest between sets)
3x30 Russian Twists (1-2 minute rest between sets)

Workout 5)

4x10 3-1 tempo Sumo Squats (lower into the movement for 3 seconds then stand up in 1) (2-3 minute rest between sets)
3x10 Dumbbell Hip Thrusts (1-2 minute rest between sets) *(replace with glute bridges if you don't want to use a bench!)*
3x10 Single Leg Dumbbell Hip Thrust (1-2 minute rest between sets)
(replace with single leg glute bridges if you don't want to use a bench!)
3x10 Dumbbell Chest Press (1-2 minute rest between sets)
3x10 Chest Flys (1-2 minute rest between sets)
3x10 Lying Leg Raise (1-2 minute rest between sets)

Workout 6)

3x10 Dumbbell Hip Thrusts (2-3 minute rest between sets) *(replace with glute bridges if you don't want to use a bench!)*
3x10 Single Leg Dumbbell Hip Thrust (1-2 minute rest between sets)
(replace with single leg glute bridges if you don't want to use a bench!)
3x10 each side Rear Foot Elevated Bulgarian Split Squat (1-2 minute rest between sets)
3x10 Dumbbell Shoulder Press (1-2 minute rest between sets)
3x10 Lateral Shoulder Raises (1-2 minute rest between sets)
3x10 Lying Leg Raise (1-2 minute rest between sets)

Workout 7)

4x10 Dumbbell Romanian Deadlift (2-3 minute rest between sets)
3x10 each side Rear Foot Elevated Bulgarian Split Squat (1-2 minute rest between sets)
3x10 each side Standing Hip Abduction (1-2 minute rest between sets)
3x10 Dumbbell Bent Over Row (1-2 minute rest between sets)
3x10 Single Arm Bent Over Row (1-2 minute rest between sets)
3x10 Lying Leg Raise (1-2 minute rest between sets)

Workout 8)

4x10 Dumbbell Romanian Deadlift (2-3 minute rest between sets)
3x10 each side Reverse Lunge (1-2 minute rest between sets)
3x10 Close Stance Dumbbell Goblet Squat (1-2 minute rest between sets)
3x10 Dumbbell Shoulder Press (1-2 minute rest between sets)
3x10 Bent Over Rear Fly (1-2 minute rest between sets)
3x10 Lying Lumbar Extension (1-2 minute rest between sets)

Workout 9)

4x10 Dumbbell Romanian Deadlift (2-3 minute rest between sets)
3x10 each side Rear Foot Elevated Bulgarian Split Squat (1-2 minute rest between sets)
3x10 each leg Single Leg Dumbbell Hip Thrust (1-2 minute rest between sets)
3x10 Push Ups (modified if needed) (1-2 minute rest between sets)
3x10 Chest Flys (1-2 minute rest between sets)
3x10 Lying Leg Raise (1-2 minute rest between sets)

Workout 10)

4x10 Dumbbell Hip Thrust (2-3 minute rest between sets) *(replace with glute bridges if you don't want to use a bench!)*
3x10 each leg Single Leg Dumbbell Hip Thrust (1-2 minute rest between sets) *(replace with single leg glute bridges if you don't want to use a bench!)*
3x10 each side Rear Foot Elevated Bulgarian Split Squat (1-2 minute rest between sets)
3x10 Dumbbell Bent Over Row (1-2 minute rest between sets)
3x10 each side Single Arm Bent Over Row (1-2 minute rest between sets)
4x30 Russian Twist (1-2 minute rest between sets)

Workout 11)

4x10 Dumbbell Hip Thrust (2-3 minute rest between sets) *(replace with glute bridges if you don't want to use a bench!)*
3x10 each leg Single Leg Dumbbell Hip Thrust (1-2 minute rest between sets) *(replace with single leg glute bridges if you don't want to use a bench!)*
3x10 each side Reverse Lunge (1-2 minute rest between sets)
3x10 Dumbbell Shoulder Press (1-2 minute rest between sets)
3x10 Lateral Shoulder Raises (1-2 minute rest between sets)
3x10 Lying Leg Raise (1-2 minute rest between sets)

Workout 12)

3x10 each side Bird Dogs (1-2 minute rest between sets)
4x10 Dumbbell Hip Thrust (2-3 minute rest between sets) *(replace with glute bridges if you don't want to use a bench!)*
3x10 each leg Single Leg Dumbbell Hip Thrust (1-2 minute rest between sets) *(replace with single leg glute bridges if you don't want to use a bench!)*
3x10 Push Ups (modified if needed) (1-2 minute rest between sets)
3x30 Russian Twists (1-2 minute rest between sets)
3x10 Lying Leg Raise (1-2 minute rest between sets)

Workout 13)

3x10 each side Bird Dogs (1-2 minute rest between sets)
4x10 Dumbbell Hip Thrust (2-3 minute rest between sets) *(replace with glute bridges if you don't want to use a bench!)*
3x10 each side Reverse Lunge (1-2 minute rest between sets)
3x10 Dumbbell Bent Over Row (1-2 minute rest between sets)
3x10 each side Single Arm Bent Over Row (1-2 minute rest between sets)
3x10 Lying Leg Raise (1-2 minute rest between sets)

Workout 14)

3x10 each side Bird Dogs (1-2 minute rest between sets)
4x10 Dumbbell Hip Thrust (2-3 minute rest between sets) *(replace with glute bridges if you don't want to use a bench!)*
3x10 each side Rear Foot Elevated Bulgarian Split Squat (1-2 minute rest between sets)
3x10 Dumbbell Shoulder Press (1-2 minute rest between sets)
3x10 Dumbbell Rear Fly (1-2 minute rest between sets)
3x10 Lateral Shoulder Raises (1-2 minute rest between sets)
3x30 Russian Twists (1-2 minute rest between sets)

Workout 15)

4x10 3-1 tempo Sumo Squats (lower into the movement for 3 seconds then stand up in 1) (2-3 minute rest between sets)
3x10 each side Single Leg Romanian Deadlifts (1-2 minute rest between sets)
3x10 each side Standing Hip Abduction (1-2 minute rest between sets)
4x10 Dumbbell Bent Over Rows (1-2 minute rest between sets)
3x10 Dumbbell Reverse Flys (1-2 minute rest between sets)
3x30 Russian Twists (1-2 minute rest between sets)
3x10 Lying Leg Raise (1-2 minute rest between sets)

Workout 16)

4x10 Dumbbell Thrusters (2-3 minute rest between sets)
3x10 Dumbbell Romanian Deadlifts (1-2 minute rest between sets)
3x10 each side Single Leg Romanian Deadlifts (1-2 minute rest between sets)
3x10 Dumbbell Shoulder Press (1-2 minute rest between sets)
3x10 Lateral Shoulder Raises (1-2 minute rest between sets)
3x30 Russian Twists (1-2 minute rest between sets)

Workout 17)

3x10 each side Bird Dogs (1-2 minute rest between sets)
4x10 Dumbbell Close Stance Sumo Squats (2-3 minute rest between sets)
3x10 each side Rear Foot Elevated Bulgarian Split Squat (1-2 minute rest between sets)
3x10 Push Ups (modified if needed) (1-2 minute rest between sets)
3x30 Russian Twists (1-2 minute rest between sets)
3x10 Lying Leg Raise (1-2 minute rest between sets)

Workout 18)

4x10 Dumbbell Thrusters (2-3 minute rest between sets)
3x10 Dumbbell Romanian Deadlifts (1-2 minute rest between sets)
3x10 each side Rear Foot Elevated Bulgarian Split Squat (1-2 minute rest between sets)
3x10 Push Ups (modified if needed) (1-2 minute rest between sets)
3x10 Dumbbell Reverse Flys (1-2 minute rest between sets)
3x10 Lying Leg Raise (1-2 minute rest between sets)

Workout 19)

4x10 Dumbbell Thrusters (2-3 minute rest between sets)

3x10 Sumo Squats (1-2 minute rest between sets)

3x10 each side Single Leg Romanian Deadlifts (1-2 minute rest between sets)

3x10 Dumbbell Bent Over Rows (1-2 minute rest between sets)

3x10 each side Single Arm Bent Over Row (1-2 minute rest between sets)

3x30 Russian Twists (1-2 minute rest between sets)

Workout 20)

4x10 3-1 tempo Dumbbell Romanian Deadlifts (3 seconds to lower into the movement, 1 second to stand up) (2-3 minute rest between sets)

3x10 each side Rear Foot Elevated Bulgarian Split Squat (1-2 minute rest between sets)

3x10 each side Single Leg Dumbbell Hip Thrust (1-2 minute rest between sets) *(replace with single leg glute bridges if you don't want to use a bench!)*

3x10 Dumbbell Chest Press (1-2 minute rest between sets)

3x10 Dumbbell Reverse Flys (1-2 minute rest between sets)

3x10 Lying Leg Raise (1-2 minute rest between sets)

Workout 21)

4x10 3-1 tempo Dumbbell Romanian Deadlifts (3 seconds to lower into the movement, 1 second to stand up) (2-3 minute rest between sets)

3x10 each side Single Leg Romanian Deadlift (1-2 minute rest between sets)

3x10 each side Standing Hip Abduction (1-2 minute rest between sets)

3x10 Dumbbell Shoulder Press (1-2 minute rest between sets)

3x10 Dumbbell Reverse Flys (1-2 minute rest between sets)

3x10 Lying Leg Raise (1-2 minute rest between sets)

Workout 22)

4x10 3-1 tempo Dumbbell Romanian Deadlifts (3 seconds to lower into the movement, 1 second to stand up) (2-3 minute rest between sets)

3x10 Dumbbell Hip Thrust (1-2 minute rest between sets) *(replace with glute bridges if you don't want to use a bench!)*

3x10 each side Single Leg Dumbbell Hip Thrust (1-2 minute rest between sets) *(replace with single leg glute bridges if you don't want to use a bench!)*

3x10 Dumbbell Shoulder Press (1-2 minute rest between sets)

3x10 Shoulder Lateral Raises (1-2 minute rest between sets)

3x10 Dumbbell Thrusters (2-3 minute rest between sets)

Workout 23)

4x10 3-1 tempo Dumbbell Romanian Deadlifts (3 seconds to lower into the movement, 1 second to stand up) (2-3 minute rest between sets)

3x1 Dumbbell Hip Thrust (1-2 minute rest between sets) *(replace with glute bridges if you don't want to use a bench!)*

3x10 each side Reverse Lunge (1-2 minute rest between sets)

3x10 Dumbbell Bent Over Rows (1-2 minute rest between sets)

3x10 each side Single Arm Bent Over Row (1-2 minute rest between sets)

3x10 Lying Leg Raises (1-2 minute rest between sets)

Workout 24)

4x10 Sumo Squats (2-3 minute rest between sets)

3x10 3-1 tempo Dumbbell Romanian Deadlifts (3 seconds to lower into the movement, 1 second to stand up) (1-2 minute rest between sets)

3x10 each side Single Leg Romanian Deadlift (1-2 minute rest between sets)

3x10 Lying Lumbar Extensions (1-2 minute rest between sets)

4x30 Russian Twists (1-2 minute rest between sets)

3x10 Lying Leg Raises (1-2 minute rest between sets)

Workout 25)

4x10 Sumo Squats (2-3 minute rest between sets)
3x10 3-1 tempo Dumbbell Romanian Deadlifts (3 seconds to lower into the movement, 1 second to stand up) (2-3 minute rest between sets)
3x10 each side Rear Foot Elevated Bulgarian Split Squat (1-2 minute rest between sets)
3x10 Dumbbell Shoulder Press (1-2 minute rest between sets)
4x30 Russian Twists (1-2 minute rest between sets)
3x10 Lying Leg Raises (1-2 minute rest between sets)

Workout 26)

3x10 each side Standing Hip Abduction (1-2 minute rest between sets)
3x10 3-1 tempo Dumbbell Romanian Deadlifts (3 seconds to lower into the movement, 1 second to stand up) (2-3 minute rest between sets)
3x10 each side Rear Foot Elevated Bulgarian Split Squat (1-2 minute rest between sets)
3x10 Bicep Curls (1-2 minute rest between sets)
3x10 Tricep Kickbacks (1-2 minute rest between sets)
4x10 Lying Leg Raises (1-2 minute rest between sets)

Workout 27)

3x10 Push Ups (modified if needed) (2-3 minute rest between sets)
3x10 each side Standing Hip Abduction (1-2 minute rest between sets)
4x10 Dumbbell Romanian Deadlifts (2-3 minute rest between sets)
3x10 each side Rear Foot Elevated Bulgarian Split Squat (1-2 minute rest between sets)
3x10 Dumbbell Chest Press (1-2 minute rest between sets)
3x10 Chest Flys (1-2 minute rest between sets)

Workout 28)

3x10 Push Ups (modified if needed) (2-3 minute rest between sets)
3x10 Dumbbell Thrusters (1-2 minute rest between sets)
3x10 each side Single Leg Romanian Deadlift (1-2 minute rest between sets)
3x10 each side Single Leg Hip Thrust (1-2 minute rest between sets)
(replace with single leg glute bridges if you don't want to use a bench!)
3x10 Lateral Shoulder Raises (1-2 minute rest between sets)
3x10 Lying Leg Raises (1-2 minute rest between sets)

Workout 29)

4x10 Dumbbell Thrusters (2-3 minute rest between sets)
3x10 each side Reverse Lunge (1-2 minute rest between sets)
3x10 Dumbbell Shoulder Press (1-2 minute rest between sets)
3x10 Bicep Curls (1-2 minute rest between sets)
3x10 Tricep Kickbacks (1-2 minute rest between sets)
4x10 Lying Leg Raises (1-2 minute rest between sets)

Workout 30)

4x10 Close Stance Dumbbell Goblet Squat (2-3 minute rest between sets)
3x10 each side Reverse Lunge (1-2 minute rest between sets)
3x10 Dumbbell Shoulder Press (1-2 minute rest between sets)
3x10 Lateral Shoulder Raises (1-2 minute rest between sets)
3x10 Bicep Curls (1-2 minute rest between sets)
3x30 Russian Twists (1-2 minute rest between sets)

Workout 31)

4x10 Standard Dumbbell Squat (2-3 minute rest between sets)
3x10 Dumbbell Romanian Deadlift (1-2 minute rest between sets)
3x10 each side Single Leg Dumbbell Romanian Deadlift (1-2 minute rest between sets)
3x10 Dumbbell Shoulder Press (1-2 minute rest between sets)
3x10 Dumbbell Bent Over Row (1-2 minute rest between sets)
3x30 Russian Twists (1-2 minute rest between sets)

Workout 32)

4x10 Standard Dumbbell Squat (2-3 minute rest between sets)
3x10 Dumbbell Hip Thrust (1-2 minute rest between sets) *(replace with glute bridges if you don't want to use a bench!)*
3x10 each side Single Leg Dumbbell Romanian Deadlift (1-2 minute rest between sets)
3x10 Dumbbell Bent Over Row (1-2 minute rest between sets)
3x10 Lying Leg Raises (1-2 minute rest between sets)
3x10 Bent Over Reverse Fly (1-2 minute rest between sets)

Workout 33)

4x10 Standard Dumbbell Squat (2-3 minute rest between sets)
3x10 Dumbbell Romanian Deadlift (1-2 minute rest between sets)
3x10 each side Rear Foot Elevated Bulgarian Split Squat (1-2 minute rest between sets)
3x10 Dumbbell Bent Over Row (1-2 minute rest between sets)
3x10 Bent Over Reverse Fly (1-2 minute rest between sets)
3x10 Squat Jumps (1-2 minute rest between sets)

Workout 34)

4x10 3-1 tempo Standard Dumbbell Squat (3 seconds to lower into the movement, 1 second to stand up) (2-3 minute rest between sets)
3x10 Dumbbell Romanian Deadlift (1-2 minute rest between sets)
3x10 each side Single Leg Dumbbell Romanian Deadlift (1-2 minute rest between sets)
3x10 Lateral Shoulder Raises (1-2 minute rest between sets)
3x10 Bicep Curls (1-2 minute rest between sets)
3x30 Russian Twists (1-2 minute rest between sets)

Workout 35)

4x10 3-1 tempo Standard Dumbbell Squat (3 seconds to lower into the movement, 1 second to stand up) (2-3 minute rest between sets)
3x10 each side Rear Foot Elevated Bulgarian Split Squat (1-2 minute rest between sets)
4x10 Dumbbell Bent Over Rows (1-2 minute rest between sets)
3x30 Russian Twists (superset) (1-2 minute rest between sets)
3x10 Lying Leg Raises (superset) (1-2 minute rest between sets)

Workout 36)

4x10 Standard Dumbbell Squat (2-3 minute rest between sets)
3x10 each side Reverse Lunge (1-2 minute rest between sets)
3x10 Dumbbell Shoulder Press (1-2 minute rest between sets)
3x10 Dumbbell Bent Over Row (1-2 minute rest between sets)
3x10 Dumbbell Lateral Shoulder Raise (1-2 minute rest between sets)
3x10 Dumbbell Reverse Fly (1-2 minute rest between sets)

Workout 37)

3x10 Squat Jumps (1-2 minute rest between sets)
4x10 Dumbbell Romanian Deadlift (2-3 minute rest between sets)
3x10 each side Dumbbell Single Leg Romanian Deadlift (1-2 minute rest between sets)
3x10 Dumbbell Shoulder Press (superset) (1-2 minute rest between sets)
3x10 Dumbbell Bent Over Row (superset) (1-2 minute rest between sets)
4x10 Lying Leg Raises(1-2 minute rest between sets)

Workout 38)

3x10 each side Bird Dogs (1-2 minute rest between sets)
3x10 Squat Jumps (1-2 minute rest between sets)
3x10 3-1 tempo Standard Dumbbell Squat (3 seconds to lower into the movement, 1 second to stand up) (2-3 minute rest between sets)
3x10 Push Ups (modified if needed) (1-2 minute rest between sets)
3x30 Russian Twists (superset) (1-2 minute rest between sets)
4x10 Lying Leg Raises (superset) (1-2 minute rest between sets)

Workout 39)

3x10 each side Bird Dogs (1-2 minute rest between sets)
3x10 Squat Jumps (1-2 minute rest between sets)
4x10 each side Reverse Lunge (1-2 minute rest between sets)
3x10 Push Ups (modified if needed) (1-2 minute rest between sets)
3x10 Chest Flys (1-2 minute rest between sets)
3x30 Russian Twists (superset) (1-2 minute rest between sets)
3x10 Lying Leg Raises (superset) (1-2 minute rest between sets)

Workout 40)

3x10 each side Bird Dogs (1-2 minute rest between sets)
3x10 Squat Jumps (1-2 minute rest between sets)
4x10 Dumbbell Romanian Deadlifts (2-3 minute rest between sets)
3x10 Push Ups (modified if needed) (1-2 minute rest between sets)
3x10 Bicep Curls (superset) (1-2 minute rest between sets)
3x10 Tricep Kickbacks (superset) (1-2 minute rest between sets)

Workout 41)

3x10 each side Bird Dogs (1-2 minute rest between sets)
3x10 3-1 tempo Dumbbell Romanian Deadlifts (3 seconds to lower into the movement, 1 second to stand up) (2-3 minute rest between sets)
3x10 Standing Hip Abduction (1-2 minute rest between sets)
3x10 Push Ups (modified if needed) (1-2 minute rest between sets)
3x10 Squat Jumps (1-2 minute rest between sets)

Workout 42)

3x10 Squat Jumps (1-2 minute rest between sets)
4x10 Dumbbell Romanian Deadlift (2-3 minute rest between sets)
3x10 each side Rear Foot Elevated Bulgarian Split Squat (1-2 minute rest between sets)
3x10 Bicep Curls (superset) (1-2 minute rest between sets)
3x10 Tricep Kickbacks (superset) (1-2 minute rest between sets)
3x30 Russian Twists (1-2 minute rest between sets)

Workout 43)

3x10 Squat Jumps (1-2 minute rest between sets)
3x10 each side bench/box Step Ups (1-2 minute rest between sets) (if you don't feel confident enough to do these, swap them with single leg dumbbell glute bridges!)
3x10 Dumbbell Shoulder Press (1-2 minute rest between sets)
3x10 Dumbbell Bent Over Row (1-2 minute rest between sets)
3x10 Dumbbell Thrusters (1-2 minute rest between sets)

Workout 44)

3x10 each side Bird Dogs (1-2 minute rest between sets)
3x10 Dumbbell Hip Thrusts (1-2 minute rest between sets) *(replace with glute bridges if you don't want to use a bench!)*
3x10 each side bench/box Step Ups (1-2 minute rest between sets) (if you don't feel confident enough to do these, swap them with single leg dumbbell glute bridges!)
3x10 Push Ups (modified if needed) (1-2 minute rest between sets)
3x30 Russian Twists (superset) (1-2 minute rest between sets)
3x10 Lying Leg Raises (superset) (1-2 minute rest between sets)

Workout 45)

3x10 each side Bird Dogs (1-2 minute rest between sets)
3x10 Dumbbell Thrusters (1-2 minute rest between sets)
3x10 each side bench/box Step Ups (1-2 minute rest between sets) (if you don't feel confident enough to do these, swap them with single leg dumbbell glute bridges!)
3x10 Dumbbell Bent Over Row (1-2 minute rest between sets)
3x10 each side Single Arm Bent Over Row (1-2 minute rest between sets)
4x10 Lying Leg Raises (1-2 minute rest between sets)

Workout 46)

3x10 each side Bird Dogs (1-2 minute rest between sets)
3x10 Dumbbell Thrusters (1-2 minute rest between sets)
3x10 Dumbbell Romanian Deadlifts (2-3 minute rest between sets)
3x10 Dumbbell Shoulder Press (1-2 minute rest between sets)
3x10 Dumbbell Chest Press (1-2 minute rest between sets)
4x10 Lying Leg Raises (1-2 minute rest between sets)

Workout 47)

3x10 Dumbbell Romanian Deadlift (2-3 minute rest between sets)
3x10 each side Single Leg Dumbbell Romanian Deadlift (1-2 minute rest between sets)
3x10 Dumbbell Bent Over Row (1-2 minute rest between sets)
3x10 each side Single Arm Bent Over Row (1-2 minute rest between sets)
3x10 Lying Lumbar Extension (1-2 minute rest between sets)
3x30 seconds Wall Sit (1-2 minute rest between sets)

Workout 48)

3x10 Dumbbell Thrusters (1-2 minute rest between sets)
3x10 Single Leg Romanian Deadlifts (1-2 minute rest between sets)
3x10 Squat Jumps (1-2 minute rest between sets)
3x10 Dumbbell Bent Over Row (1-2 minute rest between sets)
3x10 Dumbbell Chest Press (1-2 minute rest between sets)
4x10 Lying Ab Toe Taps (1-2 minute rest between sets)

Workout 49)

3x10 Dumbbell Thrusters (1-2 minute rest between sets)
3x10 Dumbbell Romanian Deadlift (2-3 minute rest between sets)
3x10 Dumbbell Bent Over Row (1-2 minute rest between sets)
3x10 each side Single Arm Bent Over Row (1-2 minute rest between sets)
3x10 Squat Jumps (1-2 minute rest between sets)
4x10 Lying Ab Toe Taps (1-2 minute rest between sets)

Workout 50)

3x10 3-1 tempo Standard Dumbbell Squats (3 seconds to lower into the movement, 1 second to stand up) (2-3 minute rest between sets)
3x10 Squat Jumps (1-2 minute rest between sets)
3x10 Dumbbell Shoulder Press (1-2 minute rest between sets)
3x10 Dumbbell Chest Press (1-2 minute rest between sets)
3x10 Lateral Shoulder Raises (1-2 minute rest between sets)
4x10 Lying Ab Toe Taps (1-2 minute rest between sets)

Workout 51)

3x10 3-1 tempo Standard Dumbbell Squats (3 seconds to lower into the movement, 1 second to stand up) (2-3 minute rest between sets)
3x10 Dumbbell Romanian Deadlift (1-2 minute rest between sets)
3x10 each side Single Arm Bent Over Row (1-2 minute rest between sets)
4x10 Dumbbell Chest Press (superset) (1-2 minute rest between sets)
4x10 Bent Over Reverse Fly (superset) (1-2 minute rest between sets)
4x10 Lying Ab Toe Taps (1-2 minute rest between sets)

Workout 52)

3x10 3-1 tempo Standard Dumbbell Squats (3 seconds to lower into the movement, 1 second to stand up) (2-3 minute rest between sets)
3x10 each side Rear Foot Elevated Bulgarian Split Squat (1-2 minute rest between sets)
3x10 Dumbbell Shoulder Press (1-2 minute rest between sets)
3x10 Bent Over Reverse Fly (superset) (1-2 minute rest between sets)
3x10 Dumbbell Upright Row (superset) (1-2 minute rest between sets)
3x30 Russian Twists (superset) (1-2 minute rest between sets)
3x10 Lying Ab Toe Taps (superset) (1-2 minute rest between sets)

Workout 53)

3x10 Dumbbell Romanian Deadlift (2-3 minute rest between sets)
3x10 Dumbbell Hip Thrust (1-2 minute rest between sets) *(replace with glute bridges if you don't want to use a bench!)*
3x10 each side 3-1 tempo Rear Foot Elevated Bulgarian Split Squat (3 seconds to lower into the movement, 1 second to stand up) (1-2 minute rest between sets)
3x10 Dumbbell Upright Row (1-2 minute rest between sets)
3x10 Bent Over Reverse Fly (1-2 minute rest between sets)
4x10 Lying Ab Toe Taps (1-2 minute rest between sets)

Workout 54)

3x10 Dumbbell Romanian Deadlift (1-2 minute rest between sets)
3x10 1 and ¼ Dumbbell Hip Thrust (2-3 minute rest between sets)
(replace with glute bridges if you don't want to use a bench!)
3x10 each side Standing Hip Abduction (1-2 minute rest between sets)
3x10 Dumbbell Bent Over Row (1-2 minute rest between sets)
3x10 Dumbbell Upright Row (1-2 minute rest between sets)
4x10 Lying Ab Toe Taps (1-2 minute rest between sets)

Workout 55)

4x10 1 and ¼ Dumbbell Hip Thrust (2-3 minute rest between sets)
(replace with glute bridges if you don't want to use a bench!)
3x10 each side Single Leg Dumbbell Hip Thrust (1-2 minute rest between sets) *(replace with single leg glute bridges if you don't want to use a bench!)*
3x10 Dumbbell Bent Over Row (1-2 minute rest between sets)
3x10 Dumbbell Upright Row (1-2 minute rest between sets)
3x10 Squat Jumps (1-2 minute rest between sets)
3x10 each side Clam Shells (1-2 minute rest between sets)

Workout 56)

4x10 1 and ¼ Dumbbell Hip Thrust (2-3 minute rest between sets)
(replace with glute bridges if you don't want to use a bench!)
3x10 each side Single Leg Dumbbell Romanian Deadlift (1-2 minute rest between sets)
3x10 Dumbbell Bent Over Row (1-2 minute rest between sets)
3x10 Dumbbell Upright Row (1-2 minute rest between sets)
3x10 Bent Over Reverse Fly (1-2 minute rest between sets)
3x10 each side Clam Shells (1-2 minute rest between sets)

Workout 57)

4x10 1 and ¼ Dumbbell Hip Thrust (2-3 minute rest between sets)
(replace with glute bridges if you don't want to use a bench!)
3x10 Rear Foot Elevated Bulgarian Split Squat (1-2 minute rest between sets)
3x10 each side Standing Hip Abduction (1-2 minute rest between sets)
3x10 each side Single Arm Bent Over Row (1-2 minute rest between sets)
3x10 Dumbbell Shoulder Press (1-2 minute rest between sets)
3x10 Bent Over Reverse Flys (1-2 minute rest between sets)
4x10 Lying Ab Toe Taps (1-2 minute rest between sets)

Workout 58)

3x10 each side Bird Dogs (1-2 minute rest between sets)
3x10 1 and ¼ Dumbbell Hip Thrust (2-3 minute rest between sets)
(replace with glute bridges if you don't want to use a bench!)
3x10 each side Single Leg Dumbbell Hip Thrust (1-2 minute rest between sets) *(replace with single leg glute bridges if you don't want to use a bench!)*
3x10 Dumbbell Shoulder Press (1-2 minute rest between sets)
3x10 Bent Over Reverse Fly (1-2 minute rest between sets)
4x10 Lying Ab Toe Taps (1-2 minute rest between sets)

Workout 59)

3x10 each side Bird Dogs (1-2 minute rest between sets)
3x10 3-1 tempo Standard Dumbbell Squats (3 seconds to lower into the movement, 1 second to stand up) (2-3 minute rest between sets)
3x10 each side Single Leg Dumbbell Romanian Deadlift (1-2 minute rest between sets)
3x10 Dumbbell Shoulder Press (1-2 minute rest between sets)
3x10 Dumbbell Bent Over Row (1-2 minute rest between sets)
4x10 Lying Ab Toe Taps (1-2 minute rest between sets)

Workout 60)

3x10 each side Bird Dogs (1-2 minute rest between sets)
3x10 3-1 tempo Sumo Squats (3 seconds to lower into the movement, 1 second to stand up) (2-3 minute rest between sets)
3x10 each side Single Leg Dumbbell Romanian Deadlift (1-2 minute rest between sets)
3x10 Dumbbell Upright Row (1-2 minute rest between sets)
3x10 Dumbbell Bent Over Row (1-2 minute rest between sets)
3x10 Lying Leg Raises (1-2 minute rest between sets)

Workout 61)

4x10 Standard Dumbbell Squat (2-3 minute rest between sets)
3x10 each side 3-1 tempo Rear Foot Elevated Bulgarian Split Squat (3 seconds to lower into the movement, 1 second to stand up) (1-2 minute rest between sets)
3x10 Dumbbell Bent Over Row (1-2 minute rest between sets)
3x10 Dumbbell Shoulder Press (1-2 minute rest between sets)
3x30 Russian Twists (superset) (1-2 minute rest between sets)
3x10 Lying Ab Toe Taps (superset) (1-2 minute rest between sets)

Workout 62)

4x10 Dumbbell Front Squat (1-2 minute rest between sets)
3x10 Dumbbell Shoulder Press (1-2 minute rest between sets)
3x10 each side Single Arm Bent Over Row (1-2 minute rest between sets)
3x10 Dumbbell Upright Row (1-2 minute rest between sets)
3x10 Squat Jumps (last set until failure) (1-2 minute rest between sets)

Workout 63)

3x10 3-1 tempo Dumbbell Front Squat (3 seconds to lower into the movement, 1 second to stand up) (2-3 minute rest between sets)
3x10 each side Reverse Lunge (1-2 minute rest between sets)
3x10 Dumbbell Shoulder Press (1-2 minute rest between sets)
3x10 Dumbbell Bent Over Row (1-2 minute rest between sets)
3x10 each side Clam Shells (1-2 minute rest between sets)
3x10 Lying Ab Toe Taps (1-2 minute rest between sets)

Workout 64)

3x10 3-1 tempo Dumbbell Front Squat (3 seconds to lower into the movement, 1 second to stand up) (2-3 minute rest between sets)
3x10 each side box/bench Step Ups (1-2 minute rest between sets) (If you don't feel confident enough to do these, replace with single leg dumbbell glute bridges!)
3x10 Dumbbell Bent Over Row (1-2 minute rest between sets)
3x10 Dumbbell Chest Press (superset) (1-2 minute rest between sets)
3x10 Dumbbell Reverse Flys (superset) (1-2 minute rest between sets)
4x10 Lying Ab Toe Taps (1-2 minute rest between sets)

Workout 65)

4x10 Dumbbell Romanian Deadlift (2-3 minute rest between sets)
3x10 Dumbbell Bent Over Row (1-2 minute rest between sets)
3x10 Single Leg Romanian Deadlifts (1-2 minute rest between sets)
3x10 each side Single Arm Bent Over Row (1-2 minute rest between sets)
3x10 Squat Jumps (1-2 minute rest between sets)
3x30 seconds Wall Sit (1-2 minute rest between sets)

Glute Focussed Workouts

Workout 1)

3x10 each side Bird Dogs (1-2 minute rest between sets)
4x10 Dumbbell Sumo Squat (2-3 minute rest between sets)
3x10 Dumbbell Romanian Deadlift (1-2 minute rest between sets)
3x10 each side Single Leg Dumbbell Romanian Deadlift (1-2 minute rest between sets)
3x10 each side Standing Hip Abduction (1-2 minute rest between sets)

Workout 2)

3x10 each side Bird Dogs (1-2 minute rest between sets)
4x10 Dumbbell Romanian Deadlift (2-3 minute rest between sets)
3x10 Dumbbell Hip Thrusts (1-2 minute rest between sets) *(replace with glute bridges if you don't want to use a bench!)*
3x10 each side Single Leg Dumbbell Hip Thrusts (1-2 minute rest between sets) *(replace with single leg glute bridges if you don't want to use a bench!)*
3x10 each side Standing Hip Abduction (1-2 minute rest between sets)

Workout 3)

3x10 each side Bird Dogs (1-2 minute rest between sets)
3x10 each side Standing Hip Abduction (1-2 minute rest between sets)
4x10 Dumbbell Hip Thrusts (2-3 minute rest between sets) *(replace with glute bridges if you don't want to use a bench!)*
3x10 Dumbbell Romanian Deadlift (1-2 minute rest between sets)
3x10 each side Single Leg Dumbbell Romanian Deadlift (1-2 minute rest between sets)

Workout 4)

3x10 each side Bird Dogs (1-2 minute rest between sets)
4x10 Dumbbell Sumo Squats (2-3 minute rest between sets)
3x10 Dumbbell Hip Thrusts (2-3 minute rest between sets) *(replace with glute bridges if you don't want to use a bench!)*
3x10 each side Rear Foot Elevated Bulgarian Split Squats (1-2 minute rest between sets)
3x10 each side Standing Hip Abduction (1-2 minute rest between sets)

Workout 5)

3x10 each side Standing Hip Abduction (1-2 minute rest between sets)
4x10 Dumbbell Hip Thrusts (2-3 minute rest between sets) *(replace with glute bridges if you don't want to use a bench!)*
3x10 each side Single Leg Dumbbell Hip Thrusts (1-2 minute rest between sets) *(replace with single leg glute bridges if you don't want to use a bench!)*
3x10 3-1 Tempo Dumbbell Sumo Squats (3 seconds to lower into the position, 1 second to stand up) (1-2 minute rest between sets)
3x10 each side Clam Shells

Workout 6)

3x10 each side Bird Dogs (1-2 minute rest between sets)
3x10 3/1 Tempo Romanian Deadlift (3 seconds to lower into the movement, 1 second to stand up) (2-3 minute rest between sets)
3x10 each side Single Leg Romanian Deadlift (1-2 minute rest between sets)
3x10 Dumbbell Glute Bridge (1-2 minute rest between sets)
3x10 each side Standing Hip Abduction (1-2 minute rest between sets)

Workout 7)

3x10 each side Bird Dogs (1-2 minute rest between sets)
4x10 3/1 Tempo Romanian Deadlift (3 seconds to lower into the movement, 1 second to stand up) (2-3 minute rest between sets)
3x10 each side Rear Foot Elevated Bulgarian Split Squat (1-2 minute rest between sets)
3x10 Dumbbell Sumo Squat (1-2 minute rest between sets)
3x10 each side Standing Hip Abduction (1-2 minute rest between sets)

Workout 8)

4x10 3/1 Tempo Romanian Deadlift (3 seconds to lower into the movement, 1 second to stand up) (2-3 minute rest between sets)
3x10 Dumbbell Sumo Squat (1-2 minute rest between sets)
3x10 each side Reverse Lunge (with a forward lean to target glutes) (1-2 minute rest between sets)
4x10 each side Clam Shell (1-2 minute rest between sets)

Workout 9)

3x10 each side Standing Hip Abduction (1-2 minute rest between sets)
4x10 3/1 Tempo Sumo Squat (3 seconds to lower into the movement, 1 second to stand up) (2-3 minute rest between sets)
3x10 each side Rear Foot Elevated Bulgarian Split Squat (1-2 minute rest between sets)
3x1 minute wall sit (1-2 minute rest between sets)
3x10 each side Clam Shell (1-2 minute rest between sets)

Workout 10)

4x10 Dumbbell Romanian Deadlift (2-3 minute rest between sets)
3x10 Dumbbell Hip Thrust (2-3 minute rest between sets) *(replace with glute bridges if you don't want to use a bench!)*
3x10 each side 3-1 Tempo Bulgarian Split Squat (3 seconds to lower into the movement, 1 second to stand up) (1-2 minute rest between sets)
3x10 each side Clam Shell (1-2 minute rest between sets)

Workout 11)

4x10 Dumbbell Romanian Deadlift (2-3 minute rest between sets)
3x10 1 and ¼ Dumbbell Hip Thrusts (2-3 minute rest between sets) *(replace with glute bridges if you don't want to use a bench!)*
3x10 each side Single Leg Hip Thrusts (1-2 minute rest between sets) *(replace with single leg glute bridges if you don't want to use a bench!)*
3x10 each side Bird Dogs (1-2 minute rest between sets)
3x10 each side Standing Hip Abduction (1-2 minute rest between sets)

Workout 12)

4x10 1 and ¼ Dumbbell Hip Thrusts (2-3 minute rest between sets) *(replace with glute bridges if you don't want to use a bench!)*
3x10 each side Single Leg Dumbbell Hip Thrust (1-2 minute rest between sets) *(replace with single leg glute bridges if you don't want to use a bench!)*
3x10 each side Single Leg Romanian Deadlifts (1-2 minute rest between sets)
3x10 each side Standing Hip Abduction (1-2 minute rest between sets)
3x10 each side Clam Shell (1-2 minute rest between sets)

Workout 13)

3x10 Dumbbell Romanian Deadlift (1-2 minute rest between sets)

3x10 Dumbbell Hip Thrusts (1-2 minute rest between sets) *(replace with glute bridges if you don't want to use a bench!)*

3x10 each side 3-1 Tempo Rear Foot Elevated Bulgarian Split Squats (3 seconds to lower into the movement, 1 second to stand up) (1-2 minute rest between sets)

3x10 each side Standing Hip Abduction (1-2 minute rest between sets)

3x30 second Wall Sit (1-2 minute rest between sets)

Lower Body Focussed Workouts

Workout 1)

3x10 Dumbbell Sumo Squats (2-3 minute rest between sets)
3x10 Close Stance Dumbbell Goblet Squats (2-3 minute rest between sets)
3x10 each side Reverse Lunge (1-2 minute rest between sets)
3x10 Squat Jumps (1-2 minute rest between sets)
3x10 each side Clam Shells (1-2 minute rest between sets)

Workout 2)

3x10 Dumbbell Thrusters (1-2 minute rest between sets)
4x10 3-1 Tempo Dumbbell Sumo Squats (3 seconds to lower into the movement, 1 second to stand up) (2-3 minute rest between sets)
3x10 each side Reverse Lunge (1-2 minute rest between sets)
3x10 Squat Jump (1-2 minute rest between sets)
3x10 each side Clam Shells (1-2 minute rest between sets)

Workout 3)

3x10 Dumbbell Thrusters (1-2 minute rest between sets)
4x10 Dumbbell Romanian Deadlift (2-3 minute rest between sets)
3x10 each side Single Leg Dumbbell Romanian Deadlift (1-2 minute rest between sets)
3x10 each side Reverse Lunge (1-2 minute rest between sets)
3x10 each side Clam Shells (1-2 minute rest between sets)

Workout 4)

3x10 Dumbbell Thrusters (1-2 minute rest between sets)
3x10 Dumbbell Romanian Deadlifts (2-3 minute rest between sets)
3x10 each side Dumbbell Single Leg Romanian Deadlift (1-2 minute rest between sets)
3x10 Squat Jumps - las set until failure (1-2 minute rest between sets)

Workout 5)

3x10 each side Dumbbell Single Leg Hip Thrusts (1-2 minute rest between sets) *(replace with single leg glute bridges if you don't want to use a bench!)*
4x10 Dumbbell Hip Thrusts (2-3 minute rest between sets) *(replace with glute bridges if you don't want to use a bench!)*
3x10 Close Stance Dumbbell Goblet Squat (1-2 minute rest between sets)
3x10 each side Reverse Lunge (1-2 minute rest between sets)
3x10 each side Standing Hip Abduction (1-2 minute rest between sets)

Workout 6)

3x10 3-1 Tempo Dumbbell Sumo Squats (3 seconds to lower into the movement, 1 second to stand up) (2-3 minute rest between sets)
3x10 each side 3-1 Tempo Bulgarian Split Squats (3 seconds to lower into the movement, 1 second to stand up) (2-3 minute rest between sets)
3x10 each side Standing Hip Abduction (1-2 minute rest between sets)
3x10 Squat Jumps (1-2 minute rest between sets)

Workout 7)

3x10 Dumbbell Thrusters (1-2 minute rest between sets)
3x10 3-1 Tempo Dumbbell Sumo Squats (3 seconds to lower into the movement, 1 second to stand up) (2-3 minute rest between sets)
3x10 each side Box Step Ups (if you're not yet confident doing this movement, perform single leg dumbbell glute bridges instead!) (1-2 minute rest between sets)
3x10 each side Standing Hip Abduction (1-2 minute rest between sets)
3x30 second Wall Sit (1-2 minute rest between sets)

Workout 8)

4x10 Dumbbell Front Squat (2-3 minute rest between sets)
3x10 Dumbbell Romanian Deadlift (1-2 minute rest between sets)
3x10 each side Box Step Ups (with dumbbells once confident with the movement) (1-2 minute rest between sets)
3x10 each side Standing Hip Abduction (1-2 minute rest between sets)
3x30 second Wall Sit (1-2 minute rest between sets)

Workout 9)

4x10 Dumbbell Front Squat (2-3 minute rest between sets)
3x10 Dumbbell Sumo Squat (1-2 minute rest between sets)
3x10 each side Rear Foot Elevated Bulgarian Split Squat (1-2 minute rest between sets)
3x10 each side Standing Hip Abduction (1-2 minute rest between sets)
3x30 second Wall Sit (1-2 minute rest between sets)

Workout 10)

4x10 Dumbbell Front Squat (2-3 minute rest between sets)

3x10 Dumbbell Hip Thrusts (1-2 minute rest between sets) *(replace with glute bridges if you don't want to use a bench!)*

3x10 each side Box Step Ups (if you're not yet confident doing these, swap for single leg dumbbell glute bridges!) (1-2 minute rest between sets)

3x10 each side Standing Hip Abduction (1-2 minute rest between sets)

3x30 second Wall Sit (1-2 minute rest between sets)

Workout 11)

4x10 Standard Dumbbell Squat (2-3 minute rest between sets)

3x10 each side Rear Foot Elevated Bulgarian Split Squat (1-2 minute rest between sets)

3x10 each side Single Leg Dumbbell Hip Thrust (1-2 minute rest between sets) *(replace with glute bridges if you don't want to use a bench!)*

3x10 each side Standing Hip Abduction (1-2 minute rest between sets)

3x30 second Wall Sit (1-2 minute rest between sets)

Workout 12)

4x10 Standard Dumbbell Squat (2-3 minute rest between sets)

3x10 Dumbbell Hip Thrusts (1-2 minute rest between sets) *(replace with glute bridges if you don't want to use a bench!)*

3x10 each side Single Leg Dumbbell Hip Thrust (1-2 minute rest between sets) *(replace with single leg glute bridges if you don't want to use a bench!)*

3x10 each side Reverse Lunge (1-2 minute rest between sets)

3x10 each side Standing Hip Abduction (1-2 minute rest between sets)

Workout 13)

4x10 Dumbbell Thrusters (2-3 minute rest between sets)
4x10 each side Rear Foot Elevated Bulgarian Split Squat (1-2 minute rest between sets)
4x10 Squat Jumps (1-2 minute rest between sets)
3x10 each side Standing Hip Abduction (1-2 minute rest between sets)

Workout 14)

4x10 Dumbbell Romanian Deadlift (2-3 minute rest between sets)
3x10 each side 3-1 Tempo Rear Foot Elevated Bulgarian Split Squats (3 seconds to lower into the movement, 1 second to stand up) (1-2 minute rest between sets)
3x10 each side Standing Hip Abduction (1-2 minute rest between sets)
3x10 Dumbbell Thrusters (1-2 minute rest between sets)
3x1 minute Wall Sit (1-2 minute rest between sets)

Workout 15)

4x10 1-3 tempo Dumbbell Hip Thrusts (1 second to thrust up, 3 seconds to lower back down) (2-3 minute rest between sets) *(replace with glute bridges if you don't want to use a bench!)*
3x10 each side Rear Foot Elevated Bulgarian Split Squats (1-2 minute rest between sets)
3x10 each side Standing Hip Abduction (1-2 minute rest between sets)
3x10 Squat Jumps (1-2 minute rest between sets)
3x1 minute Wall Sit (1-2 minute rest between sets)

Upper Body Focussed Workouts

Workout 1)

4x10 Dumbbell Bent Over Row (2-3 minute rest between sets)
3x10 each side Single Arm Dumbbell Bent Over Row (1-2 minute rest between sets)
3x10 Dumbbell Chest Press (2-3 minute rest between sets)
3x10 Chest Fly (1-2 minute rest between sets)
3x10 Bent Over Reverse Fly (1-2 minute rest between sets)

Workout 2)

4x10 Dumbbell Bent Over Row (2-3 minute rest between sets)
3x10 Dumbbell Shoulder Press (2-3 minute rest between sets)
3x10 Bent Over Reverse Fly (1-2 minute rest between sets)
3x10 Shoulder Lateral Raises (1-2 minute rest between sets)
3x10 each side Single Arm Dumbbell Bent Over Row (1-2 minute rest between sets)
3x10 Lying Ab Toe Taps (1-2 minute rest between sets)

Workout 3)

4x10 Dumbbell Chest Press (2-3 minute rest between sets)
4x10 Dumbbell Bent Over Row (2-3 minute rest between sets)
3x10 Chest Fly (1-2 minute rest between sets)
3x10 each side Single Arm Bent Over Row (1-2 minute rest between sets)
3x10 Lying Leg Raises (superset) (1-2 minute rest between sets)
3x30 Russian Twists (superset) (1-2 minute rest between sets)

Workout 4)

4x10 Dumbbell Shoulder Press (2-3 minute rest between sets)
4x10 Dumbbell Bent Over Row (2-3 minute rest between sets)
3x10 Shoulder Lateral Raises (1-2 minute rest between sets)
3x10 Bent Over Reverse Fly (1-2 minute rest between sets)
3x10 Dumbbell Thrusters (1-2 minute rest between sets)

Workout 5)

4x10 Dumbbell Bent Over Row (2-3 minute rest between sets)
3x10 Shoulder Lateral Raises (2-3 minute rest between sets)
3x10 Bent Over Reverse Fly (1-2 minute rest between sets)
4x10 Dumbbell Shoulder Press (1-2 minute rest between sets)
3x10 Lumbar Extensions (1-2 minute rest between sets)
3x10 Lying Ab Toe Taps (1-2 minute rest between sets)

Workout 6)

4x10 Dumbbell Shoulder Press (2-3 minute rest between sets)
3x10 Dumbbell Chest Press (2-3 minute rest between sets)
3x10 Dumbbell Shoulder Lateral Raises (1-2 minute rest between sets)
3x10 Dumbbell Chest Flys (1-2 minute rest between sets)
3x10 Lying Lumbar Extensions (1-2 minute rest between sets)
3x30 Russian Twists (1-2 minute rest between sets)

Workout 7)

4x10 Dumbbell Bent Over Row (2-3 minute rest between sets)
3x10 each side Single Arm Bent Over Row (1-2 minute rest between sets)
4x10 Lying Leg Raises (1-2 minute rest between sets)
3x10 Bent Over Reverse Fly (1-2 minute rest between sets)
3x10 Lying Lumbar Extensions (1-2 minute rest between sets)
3x30 Russian Twists (1-2 minute rest between sets)

Workout 8)

4x10 Dumbbell Thrusters (2-3 minute rest between sets)
3x10 Lateral Shoulder Raise (1-2 minute rest between sets)
3x10 Bicep Curl (superset) (1-2 minute rest between sets)
3x10 Tricep Kickback (superset) (1-2 minute rest between sets)
3x10 Lying Leg Raises (1-2 minute rest between sets)
3x30 Russian Twists (1-2 minute rest between sets)

Workout 9)

4x10 Dumbbell Thrusters (2-3 minute rest between sets)
4x10 Dumbbell Chest Press (2-3 minute rest between sets)
3x10 Bicep Curl (superset) (1-2 minute rest between sets)
3x10 Tricep Kickback (superset) (1-2 minute rest between sets)
3x10 Chest Flys (1-2 minute rest between sets)
3x30 Russian Twists (1-2 minute rest between sets)

Workout 10)

3x10 Push Ups (modified if needed) (1-2 minute rest between sets)
3x10 Dumbbell Shoulder Press (1-2 minute rest between sets)
3x10 each side Single Arm Bent Over Row (1-2 minute rest between sets)
3x10 Lying Lumbar Extensions (1-2 minute rest between sets)
3x10 Bent Over Reverse Fly (1-2 minute rest between sets)
3x30 Russian Twists (1-2 minute rest between sets)

Workout 11)

3x10 Dumbbell Thrusters (1-2 minute rest between sets)
3x10 Push Ups (modified if needed) (1-2 minute rest between sets)
3x10 Chest Flys (1-2 minute rest between sets)
3x10 Lateral Shoulder Raises (1-2 minute rest between sets)
3x30 Russian Twists (superset) (1-2 minute rest between sets)
3x10 Lying Leg Raises (superset) (1-2 minute rest between sets)

Workout 12)

3x10 Push Ups (modified if needed) (1-2 minute rest between sets)
4x10 Dumbbell Bent Over Row (2-3 minute rest between sets)
4x10 Dumbbell Shoulder Press
3x10 each side Single Arm Bent Over Row (1-2 minute rest between sets)
4x10 Lying Ab Toe Taps (1-2 minute rest between sets)

Workout 13)

4x10 Dumbbell Bent Over Row (2-3 minute rest between sets)
4x10 Dumbbell Chest Press (2-3 minute rest between sets)
3x10 each side Single Arm Bent Over Row (1-2 minute rest between sets)
3x10 Chest Fly (1-2 minute rest between sets)
3x10 Lying Ab Toe Taps (superset) (1-2 minute rest between sets)
3x30 Russian Twists (superset) (1-2 minute rest between sets)

Workout 14)

4x10 Dumbbell Bent Over Row (2-3 minute rest between sets)
4x10 Dumbbell Chest Press (2-3 minute rest between sets)
3x10 Dumbbell Reverse Flys (1-2 minute rest between sets)
4x10 Push Ups (modified if needed) (1-2 minute rest between sets)
3x10 Lying Ab Toe Taps (superset) (1-2 minute rest between sets)
3x30 Russian Twists (superset) (1-2 minute rest between sets)

Workout 15)

3x10 Push Ups (modified if needed) (1-2 minute rest between sets)
4x10 Dumbbell Bent Over Row (2-3 minute rest between sets)
3x10 Dumbbell Chest Press (1-2 minute rest between sets)
3x10 Bent Over Reverse Fly (1-2 minute rest between sets)
3x30 Russian Twists (superset) (1-2 minute rest between sets)
3x10 Lying Leg Raises (superset) (1-2 minute rest between sets)

Workout 16)

3x10 Push Ups (modified if needed) (1-2 minute rest between sets)
4x10 Dumbbell Bent Over Row (2-3 minute rest between sets)
3x10 each side Single Arm Bent Over Row (1-2 minute rest between sets)
3x10 Dumbbell Upright Row (1-2 minute rest between sets)
3x10 Lateral Shoulder Raise (1-2 minute rest between sets)
3x10 Lying Ab Toe Taps (1-2 minute rest between sets)

Workout 17)

3x10 Dumbbell Thrusters (1-2 minute rest between sets)
4x10 Dumbbell Chest Press (2-3 minute rest between sets)
3x10 Dumbbell Upright Row (1-2 minute rest between sets)
3x10 Chest Fly (1-2 minute rest between sets)
3x10 Lying Ab Toe Taps (superset) (1-2 minute rest between sets)
3x30 Russian Twists (superset) (1-2 minute rest between sets)

Workout 18)

4x10 Dumbbell Bent Over Row (2-3 minute rest between sets)
4x10 Dumbbell Upright Row (1-2 minute rest between sets)
3x10 each side Single Arm Bent Over Row (1-2 minute rest between sets)
3x10 Dumbbell Shoulder Press (2-3 minute rest between sets)
3x10 Bent Over Reverse Flys (1-2 minute rest between sets)
4x10 Lying Ab Toe Taps (1-2 minute rest between sets)

Part Three
Movement Glossary

Movement Glossary

Standard Dumbbell Squat:

Step 1) Hold a dumbbell in each hand and keep your hands by your side. Stand with your feet slightly wider than shoulder width apart. Take a deep breath in as you brace your core, imagining pushing your tummy out in all directions making a firm wall.

Step 2) Perform the squat by bending your knees as your body moves towards the floor as if you're going to sit on a chair. Only go as far as you can before your lower back starts to curve (this is called a butt wink - to be avoided!). Aim for your thighs to be at least parallel to the floor.

Step 3) On an exhale, push through your feet to stand back up before repeating more repetitions.

Watch a demo of this movement here:

Dumbbell Close Stance Goblet Squat:

Step 1) Hold a dumbbell with both of your hands at chest height. Place your feet together or at least closer together than shoulder width apart with your toes facing forward. Take a deep breath in as you brace your core, imagining pushing your tummy out in all directions making a firm wall.

Step 2) Sit your hips back and squat as low as you can. Only go as far as you can before your lower back starts to curve (this is called a butt wink - to be avoided!). Aim for your thighs to be at least parallel to the floor

Step 3) Exhale as you press through your feet to return to the starting position before repeating more repetitions.

Watch a demo of this movement here:

Dumbbell Sumo Squat:

Step 1) Hold a dumbbell with both of your hands keeping your arms straight down in front of your body. Stand with your feet spread wide apart and your toes pointing slightly outwards. Take a deep breath in as you brace your core, imagining pushing your tummy out in all directions making a firm wall.

Step 3) Lower your hips and bend your knees to take you into a wide squat position until your thighs are at least parallel to the floor and the dumbbell is on or near to the floor.

Step 4) Exhale as you push up through your feet and squeeze your glutes to get you back into the starting position before repeating more repetitions.

Watch a demo of this movement here:

Dumbbell Front Squat:

Step 1) Stand with your feet shoulder width apart and hold a dumbbell in each hand. Bend at the elbows so that the dumbbells are touching your shoulders, then point your elbows out in front of you so that the backs of your upper arms are parallel to the floor. Engage your core by taking a big deep breath to harden the outer layer of your stomach.

Step 3) Bend your knees to move into the squat position until your thighs are at least parallel with the floor.

Step 4) On an exhale, straighten your legs to return to standing and repeat!

Watch a demo of this movement here:

Squat Jump:

Step 1) Stand with your feet shoulder width apart and your core engaged.

Step 2) Bend your knees to lower into a squat position.

Step 3) Push through your feet to jump up off the ground using as much power as possible, before returning into the squat position to complete the rep.

Watch a demo of this movement here:

Rear Foot Elevated Bulgarian Split Squat:

Step 1) Hold a dumbbell in each hand (if desired) and stand with your feet shoulder width apart.

Step 2) Bend one of your knees, lifting the foot off the ground and placing it behind you on a bench or other elevated stable surface. The top of your foot should rest on the bench with the knee of this leg remaining bent.

Step 3) Perform a lunge with the other leg, by bending the leg as you lower towards the floor.

Step 4) Push through the active legs' foot to return to the standing position. Repeat for your desired number of reps before swapping legs.

Watch a demo of this movement here:

Dumbbell Thruster:

Step 1) Stand with your feet slightly wider than shoulder width apart and a dumbbell in each hand, with your arms down by your side. Bend your arms to bring the dumbbells in line with your shoulders.

Step 2) Perform a squat, keeping the dumbbells where they are as you move down towards the floor.

Step 3) Stand up from the squat, using the momentum to press the dumbbells up above your head when you reach the standing position.

Step 4) Lower the dumbbells back to shoulder height to finish the repetition.

Watch a demo of this movement here:

Dumbbell Romanian Deadlift:

Step 1) Hold a dumbbell in each hand and stand with your feet shoulder-width apart with a slight bend in your knees. Your feet should be pointed forward and your arms placed down in front of your body. Pull your shoulder blades back together.

Step 2) Keeping your knees slightly bent, slowly hinge your body forward, pushing your hips back as far as you can whilst lowering the dumbbells down until your back is parallel with the floor. Maintain a straight and engaged back and straight arms. Aim to keep the dumbbells as close to the fronts of the legs as possible, in line with your shoelaces. Keep your head in line with your spine.

Step 3) Keeping the muscles in your back, glutes and hamstrings engaged, pull the weight back up to the starting position.

Watch a demo of this movement here:

Single Leg Dumbbell Romanian Deadlift:

Step 1) Hold a dumbbell in each hand and stand with your feet shoulder-width apart with a slight bend in your knees. Your feet should be pointed forward and your arms placed down and in front of your body. Pull your shoulder blades back together.

Step 2) As you slowly lift one foot off the ground, keep your knees slightly bent and slowly hinge your body forward, pushing your hips backwards as far as you can and lowering the dumbbells down towards the floor until your back is parallel with the floor.

Step 3) Using control and back/hamstring/glute strength of the working leg, pull the weight back up to the starting position and place your lifted foot back on the ground for stability.

Step 4) Repeat for your desired number of repetitions before performing the movement on the other leg!

Watch a demo of this movement here:

Dumbbell Hip Thrust:

Step 1) Set up a gym bench and grab a dumbbell. Place your shoulder blades on the bench and your feet firmly on the floor shoulder hip width apart, creating a straight line from your chest to your knees, with your body parallel to the floor. Hold the dumbbell on the front of your hips (place a jumper underneath the dumbbell if this is uncomfortable).

Step 2) Keep your focus to the front with your chin tucked slightly towards your chest, don't tilt your head backwards in this movement. Take a deep breath to brace your core (to help avoid any overarching in your lower back). Lower your hips towards the floor.

Step 3) Push your feet into the floor as you push your hips back up towards the ceiling, re-forming the straight line from your chest to your knees. Hold for a second to feel the tension in your glutes. Repeat!

Watch a demo of this movement here:

Single Leg Dumbbell Hip Thrust:

Step 1) Set up a gym bench and grab a dumbbell. Place your shoulder blades on the bench and your feet firmly on the floor shoulder width apart, creating a straight line from your chest to your knees, with your body parallel to the floor. Hold the dumbbell on the front of your hips (place a jumper underneath the dumbbell if this is uncomfortable).

Step 2) Lift one foot off the ground and keep your hips straight.

Step 3) Keep your focus to the front with your chin tucked slightly towards your chest, don't tilt your head backwards in this movement. Take a deep breath to brace your core (to help avoid any overarching in your lower back) then lower your hips towards the floor, keeping one foot off the ground.

Step 4) Push your working foot into the floor as you push your hips back up towards the ceiling. Hold for a second to feel the tension in your glutes. Repeat!

Watch a demo of this movement here:

Glute Bridge:

Step 1) Lie on the floor with your knees bent and feet flat on the ground. Place your hands down on either side of your body and pull your belly button in towards your spine to engage the core. If you'd like to add some resistance, place a dumbbell on your hips.

Step 2) Squeeze the glute muscles as you lift your hips and torso off the floor until your thighs and torso are in a diagonal line. Keep your core engaged and don't overarche your back. Hold this position for a couple of seconds.

Step 3) Slowly lower under back down to the starting position and repeat!

Watch a demo of this movement here:

Reverse Lunge:

Step 1) Stand with your feet shoulder width apart and a dumbbell in each hand if desired.

Step 2) Move one leg backwards, lifting it slightly off the floor to place it behind you as you bend the knee of the acting leg to perform a lunge. Lunge until both knees are at a 90 degree angle.

Step 3) Straighten your legs as you return to standing, bringing the back leg forwards in line with the supporting leg.

Step 4) Repeat on the same leg for your desired number of repetitions before repeating the movement on the other leg.

Watch a demo of this movement here:

Wall Sit:

Step 1) Stand with your back and the backs of your feet against a wall.

Step 2) Walk your feet out in front of you to allow your body to get into a seated position with your back straight against the wall and your knees parallel to the floor.

Step 3) Hold this position for your desired number of seconds before returning to the standing position. You can hold weights in your hands or have them placed on your legs when in the seated position to add resistance to this movement.

Watch a demo of this movement here:

Box/Bench Step Up:

Step 1) Face a plyometric box or weight bench and stand a few inches away from it, with your feet shoulder width apart. If comfortable with the movement you could hold a dumbbell in each hand to add some resistance.

Step 2) Lift one foot off the ground to stand onto the box/bench, pushing the weight through the acting foot, not through the supporting one. If you lean forward slightly you should feel the resistance mostly through the glute of the acting leg.

Step 3) After standing up straight on one leg on the box/bench, lower the supporting leg back down to the ground, followed by the acting leg.

Step 4) Repeat on the same leg for your desired number of repetitions before repeating on the other leg.

Watch a demo of this movement here:

Standing Hip Abduction:

Step 1) Stand with your feet shoulder width apart with your toes facing forwards. Hold a dumbbell in one hand, with both hands resting by the sides of the body (alternatively, you could place a resistance band around your legs if you have one, below the knees).

Step 2) Hold onto a stable surface with one hand for balance, standing sideways to the surface. The hand holding the dumbbell should be resting on the outside of the opposite leg.

Step 3) Laterally raise the leg with the dumbbell against it in a slow, controlled motion. Keep your toes on this leg pointed slightly inwards and pause for one second when the leg is extended out to the side to feel the resistance in the side of the glute.

Step 4) Bring the leg back in towards the supporting leg to complete the rep. Repeat for your desired number of reps before performing the movement on the other leg.

Watch a demo of this movement here:

Clam Shells:

Step 1) Lie on your side with your knees slightly bent and your bottom arm in a comfortable position that allows you to remain stable. Keep your feet together throughout the entire movement.

Step 2) Press your bottom leg firmly into the floor and with the inside of your feet pressed together, squeeze your glute muscles to raise your top knee towards the ceiling, imagining a clam shell opening up. Move the outside knee as high as possible without letting your pelvis rock backward or forwards. Pause here for a moment, before lowering the knee back into the starting position.

Step 3) Repeat for your chosen amount of reps then lie on the opposite side and repeat on the other leg. You can add a resistance band around your legs, just above your knees if you'd like to add some more resistance to this movement.

Watch a demo of this movement here:

Bird Dogs:

Step 1) Get into a four point kneeling 'tabletop' position by placing your hands and knees on the floor. Pull your belly button in towards your spine and engage your core.

Step 2) Slide one leg backwards as far as is comfortable, stop when the leg is straight and lift the leg off the ground until it's in line with the back. Lift the opposite arm out in front of you and perform a superman arm position. Hold the leg and arm in this extended position for one second (or for up to 5 seconds if you'd like a challenge!), before returning them to the starting position.

Step 3) Repeat for your desired number of repetitions before repeating on the opposite arm and leg.

Watch a demo of this movement here:

Bicep Curl:

Step 1) Stand with your feet shoulder width apart with a dumbbell in each hand. Your arms should be down by your side with the palms of your hands facing forwards and your forearms extended.

Step 2) Bend your elbows to bring the dumbbells in to touch the top of your arms in a controlled motion. Once you reach the top of the movement, slowly lower the dumbbells down to the starting position, feeling the resistance in your biceps. Repeat!

Watch a demo of this movement here:

Tricep Kickback:

Step 1) Stand with your feet shoulder-width apart and hold a dumbbell in each hand. Bend your elbows to bring the dumbbells in line with your shoulders, with your thumbs facing your body.

Step 2) Keep your back straight as you hinge your upper body forward, keeping a slight bend in your knees.

Step 3) Engage your tricep muscles as you straighten your arms backwards by opening at the elbows. Keep your upper arms in the same position throughout. Hold this extended arm position for 2 seconds before bending your elbows to bring your arms back to the starting position. Repeat for your desired number of repetitions and stand up fully to finish.

Watch a demo of this movement here:

Push Ups:

Step 1) Get into a table top position by getting onto your hands and knees on the floor. Pull your belly button in towards your spine to engage your core.

Step 2) Move your feet back as you straighten your legs to get into the plank position. Your arms should be holding you off the floor but not fully locked out at the elbow.

Step 3) Bend your elbows to bring your body towards the floor.

Step 4) Straighten your elbows (but avoid locking them out fully!), to bring you back into the plank position. This completes the rep! Repeat for your desired number of reps.

Watch a demo of this movement here:

Variations of push ups if you can't yet perform a standard one:

Wall Push Ups:

Step 1) Place your hands shoulder width apart against a solid wall with your feet apart and weight naturally under the body.

Step 2) Bend your elbows to bring your body towards the wall as far as you feel comfortable. Straighten the arms again to push away from the wall. This completes the rep! Repeat for your desired number of reps.

Watch a demo of this movement here:

Knee Push Ups:

Step 1) Get into a tabletop position on the floor by getting onto your hands and knees. Pull your belly button in towards your spine and engage your core.

Step 2) Move your weight forwards into your hands and take your feet off the floor so that only your knees and hands are on the floor.

Step 3) Bend your elbows to bring your body closer to the floor, then push away from the floor, straightening your arms (but never fully locking out your elbows!) to finish the rep. Repeat for your desired number of reps.

Dumbbell Chest Press:

Step 1) Holding a dumbbell in each hand, lie flat on your back on a bench, with your feet flat on the floor. (If there are no benches available you can just lie on the floor with your feet on the floor and your knees bent).

Step 2) Tuck your shoulder blades back together and press down into the floor with your feet to create a small arch in your back! Your bodyweight should be resting on your glutes and shoulder blades.

Step 3) Raise your dumbbells above your head by straightening your arms.

Step 4) Lower the dumbbells to just above chest level in a controlled motion by bending your elbows (or as far down as the floor allows if doing these without a bench).

Step 5) Then press the weight back up to repeat!

Watch a demo of this movement here:

Chest Fly:

Step 1) Holding a dumbbell in each hand, lie flat on your back on a bench, with your feet flat on the floor. (If there are no benches available you can just lie on the floor with your feet on the floor and your knees bent).

Step 2) Bring your hands together above your body with your wrists facing each other. Tuck your shoulder blades back together and press down into the floor with your feet to create a small arch in your back! Your bodyweight should be resting on your glutes and shoulder blades.

Step 3) Open your hands away from each other in a controlled motion to feel the resistance in your chest muscles. Once the hands reach your shoulder line, bring them back together, don't take them lower than your shoulders. Repeat!

Watch a demo of this movement here:

Dumbbell Shoulder Press:

Step 1) Stand with your feet shoulder width apart or sit on a bench and hold a dumbbell in each hand. Lift the dumbbells up so that your upper arms are in line with your shoulders to the sides of your body. There should be a bend in your elbows with the dumbbells pointing up towards the ceiling.

Step 2) Push the dumbbells up above your head in a controlled manner until your arms extend fully (but don't lock out your elbows!). Hold the weight overhead for a second, then lower the dumbbells back to the starting height. Repeat!

Watch a demo of this movement here:

Lateral Shoulder Raise:

Step 1) Stand tall with your feet shoulder-width apart and hold a dumbbell in each hand with your arms down by your side. Pull your shoulder blades back together and engage your core.

Step 2) Raise your arms simultaneously out to the side until they're parallel with the floor, keeping a slight bend in the elbows. Pause for a moment, then lower the weights down slowly to return to the starting position.

Watch a demo of this movement here:

Standing Upright Row:

Step 1) Stand with your feet shoulder width apart and a dumbbell in each hand with your arms straight down in front of your body (the dumbbells can be touching the front of your thighs).

Step 2) Pull the dumbbells up towards your chest line, bending your elbows and keeping your core engaged and shoulder blades pulled back together. Try to not shrug your shoulders when pulling the weight up and don't move your elbows above your shoulders.

Step 3) After holding this position for a moment, move the dumbbells back down to the starting position. Repeat!

Watch a demo of this movement here:

Dumbbell Bent Over Row:

Step 1) Hold a dumbbell in each hand and stand with your feet shoulder width apart. Slightly bend your knees and hinge your upper body forwards whilst keeping your back straight. Your body should be almost parallel to the floor and your arms should be extended straight down with the dumbbells pointing towards the floor.

Step 2) Squeeze your shoulder blades back together and bend your elbows to lift the dumbbells up in line with each side of your body whilst keeping your torso still. Squeeze the shoulder blades for a moment here before slowly lowering the dumbbells back to the starting position. Repeat!

Watch a demo of this movement here:

Single Arm Dumbbell Bent Over Row:

Step 1) Hold a dumbbell in one hand and put the opposite hand and knee on a bench, bending your upper body over so that your back is straight and your body is parallel to the floor. The arm holding your dumbbell should be extended straight down towards the floor.

Step 2) Pull the shoulder blade of the arm you're holding the dumbbell with back as you bend the elbow of that arm to bring the dumbbell in line with your body. Squeeze the shoulder blade in this position for a moment before slowly lowering the dumbbell back down towards the floor. Repeat for your desired number of reps before performing on the other side.

Watch a demo of this movement here:

Lying Lumbar Extension:

Step 1) Lie on your stomach on an exercise mat or soft floor. Place your forearms on the ground next to your head with your elbows bent. Gently pull your shoulders back together.

Step 2) Press your hands into the floor as you slowly lift your upper back off the floor, without overarching. Keep your neck and head neutral. Hold this position for 10-30 seconds as you take deep breaths. Lower to the starting position then repeat. Once you're confident with this movement, you could try lifting your hands off the floor when you extend.

Watch a demo of this movement here:

Reverse Fly:

Step 1) Hold a dumbbell in each hand and stand with your feet shoulder width apart. Slightly bend your knees and hinge your upper body forwards whilst keeping your back straight. Your body should be almost parallel to the floor and your arms should be extended down with the dumbbells pointing towards the floor and the hands almost touching.

Step 2) Pull your shoulder blades together as you move the dumbbells away from each other. Pull them apart until you're forming a T shape with your upper body (but with your elbows slightly bent!). Don't move your arms any higher up than your back. Hold this position for a moment before returning to the starting position. Repeat!

Watch a demo of this movement here:

Russian Twist:

Step 1) Sit down on the floor (on a mat if you can!) and hold a dumbbell with both hands.

Step 2) Lean back slightly and lift your feet off the ground whilst bending your knees so that all of your weight is on your glutes. Keep your core engaged and back straight as you hold the dumbbell in front of your body.

Step 3) Keeping your core strong and stable, move the dumbbell to the left, then right, tapping it on the floor if you can. Repeat!

Watch a demo of this movement here:

Lying Leg Raise:

Step 1) Lie down on the floor or on a gym mat. Bend at the hips and bring your legs up to form a 90 degree angle with your legs and body.

Step 2) Keeping your hands either side of your body for stability, slowly move your legs down towards the floor, allowing your core to resist them falling. Make sure you don't arch your back!

Step 3) Bring the legs back up to form the 90 degree angle and repeat!

Watch a demo of this movement here:

Lying Ab Toe Taps:

Step 1) Lie down on the floor or on a gym mat. Bend at the hips and bring your legs up straight to form a 90 degree angle with your legs and body.

Step 2) With your arms extended above you, reach up to try and touch your toes. Keep your focus neutral. Once you've reached as far up as you can, place your body back on the ground before repeating for your desired number of reps. Once you're comfortable with this movement you could try holding a dumbbell with both hands to add some resistance.

Watch a demo of this movement here:

Congratulations!

Your transformation from shy gym girl to confident gym goddess is well underway! I hope that this book has provided you with the foundations you needed to feel comfortable in the gym, even if it's in the corner with some dumbbells for now!

We must all start somewhere and the fact that you're stepping in a gym, or even working out at home, is something to feel really proud of! With time and consistency you will see changes in your body and mindset that will have you feeling incredible and I can't wait for you to feel the pride and excitement that comes with that!

Remember that you are capable of whatever you set your mind (and body) to. Strength training and fitness in general doesn't need to be complicated and I hope if nothing else that this book has given you the tools you need to stop feeling lost in your workouts.

Well done for showing up and I wish you so much strength, happiness and confidence!

A Quick Note!

If you enjoyed this book I would be incredibly grateful if you could leave a review on Amazon.

This is free and shouldn't take any longer than 60 seconds. Reviews really help independent authors like myself get in front of the right audience and reach more people!

Thank you so much in advance!

Join our Community!

It can be isolating and daunting getting into the gym and fitness in general by yourself, so I'd like to invite you to join a community of women who support and motivate each other online (and hopefully one day in person!).

Just email 'Community' to sophie@strongandstretchy.co.uk and I'll add you into the free Facebook group!

I can't wait for you to join our supportive family!

X

Nutrition Calculations

If you're visiting this page it means you really want to take control of your nutrition and make sure you're hitting your fitness goals - good on you!! This section may seem a little overwhelming at first but once you're used to the calculations you will always be able to work out how many calories you need to consume to hit your goals.

To work this out, you'll firstly need to calculate your **total daily energy expenditure.** This is how much energy you burn every day through eating, exercising, moving and just living! Once you know what this number is, you can ensure you're consuming enough energy through your diet to either exceed it (if you want to gain muscle/weight), or eat just below it (if you want to lose weight), or eat just on it if you want to maintain your weight and just workout for fun! *Flick back to the 'Rocket Fuel' section on page 9 if you'd like a reminder of how you should approach your calorie intake depending on your goal. If you know your goal, let's jump right into the calculations!*

Firstly, it's time to work out your **total daily energy expenditure**. This can be calculated by combining four numbers - your basal metabolic rate, thermic effect of feeding, exercise energy expenditure, and non-exercise activity thermogenesis (stick with me!)

- **Your Basal Metabolic Rate (BMR)** is the number of calories your body needs to keep your organs functioning and you alive. The easiest way to calculate this is by using a machine in your gym like an InBody. But if that's not accessible to you you can calculate it using the Harris-Benedict equation, which combines your age, weight and height.
  For women the calculation is: BMR = 655.1 + (9.563 x weight in kg) + (1.850 x height in cm) - (4.676 x age in years)

Work out yours and write it down here!

- **Next is The Thermic Effect of Feeding (TEF)**, which is the energy it takes to digest your food. To calculate this just multiply your BMR by 0.1.

Work out yours and write it down here!

- The third factor contributing to your total daily energy expenditure is **Exercise Energy Expenditure (EEE).** This is the amount of energy you expend during exercise. This factor can't be calculated completely accurately as it's unique to each person based on weight, age, exercise intensity and other factors, but general guidance is that it can range from 250 calories for a gentle workout to 500 for a vigorous workout. If you have the means to buy a fitness watch, that would give you the most accurate estimate of your EEE.

But let's look at an example:

If a healthy woman who is relatively in shape and not overweight works out with medium intensity for an hour, their EEE on a typical workout day could be around 350.

Now make a rough estimate of your EEE based on the workout you typically do or will do on a normal day and write it down here!

- The fourth factor to take into account is **NEAT - Non Exercise Activity Thermogenesis.** This is the number of calories burned in everyday life outside of your workouts, eating and sleeping, when walking to work, sitting at your desk, working a physical job, performing your daily shower concert etc.. Just by using those different examples it's easy to see why NEAT can't easily be precisely calculated and you'd get the best estimation through a fitness watch as your days likely vary in terms of activeness. But NEAT typically ranges from 250 calories upwards. In fact, research biologist Cathy Koltz suggests that on average, a person's NEAT is around 300 but that this could go up to 700 or more!

Let's look at an Example:

If someone is fairly sedentary, they work a desk job and only walk to and from the kitchen, bathroom or car, their NEAT could sit around 200. If they were a construction worker it could be closer to 500 (this is a rough estimation!)

Now make a rough estimate of your NEAT levels based on your non-exercise activity on a typical day and write it down here!

Let's bring it all together!

Phew, *we're almost there!* To find your Total Daily Energy Expenditure, add all of the above together.

BMR =

TEF =

EEE =

NEAT =

(TDEE = BMR+TEF+EEE+NEAT)

Now work out your TDEE and write it here:

Whatever number you have here is the amount of calories you should consume each day to <u>maintain</u> your weight level based on the amount of

energy you expend each day through living, eating, moving and working out.

According to Legion Athletics, if you eat just ten percent more calories than you burn everyday you could gain almost as much muscle as you would if you were eating twenty or thirty percent. Ofcourse you'd also need to be consuming sufficient protein (between 0.8-1.2g per lbs of bodyweight), but with some small changes you could really see a big impact over time.

Refer back to the 'Rocket Fuel' section if you're unsure on how to approach your calorie intake depending on your goal - but here are some places to start for the most common goals of losing weight or gradually building muscle:

A good place to start if you're looking to **gradually build muscle without gaining too much fat**, would be to consume an extra 10% calories of your daily TDEE as well as between 0.8-1g of protein per pound of bodyweight. Start small and adjust as you progress.

A good place to start if you're looking to **lose weight** would be to consume between 20-35% less calories than your total TDEE, keeping your protein high to keep you full and prevent muscle loss.

What is your new daily calorie and protein goal?

Disclaimer!

It's important to note that this number can never be 100% accurate as factors such as metabolism, gender, age and height all play into the above calculations, as well as the fact that some days we move more than others. I'd always recommend speaking with a nutritionist to get the most accurate nutritional goals. Nevertheless *this math session has hopefully helped you to calculate a good calorie target to work off which is a huge step forward in your fitness journey.*

As you progress in your strength training programme you'll figure out what works best for you calorie and protein wise and can adjust the more you get to know your body.

Glossary

Resources

- Independent, T. (2019, September 9). *A quarter of women avoid exercise in fear of being judged, poll claims*. The Independent. https://www.independent.co.uk/news/health/women-sport-exercise-embarrassment-gym-anxiety-a9098021.html

- The Editors of Women's Health. (2022, April 21). *Narrow-Stance Goblet Squat*. Women's Health. https://www.womenshealthmag.com/health/a20700183/narrow-stance-goblet-squat/

- *NCBI - WWW Error Blocked Diagnostic*. (n.d.). https://pubmed.ncbi.nlm.nih.gov/27102172/ https://pubmed.ncbi.nlm.nih.gov/27102172/#:~:text=It%20can%20therefore%20be%20inferred,protocol%20remains%20to%20be%20determined.

- Origym. (2021, December 10). *The Importance of Rest Days & How Many You Need*. https://origympersonaltrainercourses.co.uk/blog/rest-days

- Women's Health Editors. (2022, May 7). *Here's How Often You Should Work Out Based On Your Goals, According To Trainers*. Women's Health. https://www.womenshealthmag.com/fitness/a35845434/how-often-should-you-workout/

- *Calorie Deficit Calculator to Lose Weight*. (n.d.). https://www.fitwatch.com/calculator/calorie-deficit

- Legion Athletics, Inc. (2021, July 26). *Calorie Calculator for Weight Loss*. Legion Athletics. https://legionathletics.com/tools/calorie-calculator/

- *Aerobic exercise: How to warm up and cool down*. (2021, October 6). Mayo Clinic. https://www.mayoclinic.org/healthy-lifestyle/fitness/in-depth/exercise/art-20045517?reDate=28112022

- Fell, J. (2018, June 17). *NEAT way to get in shape*. Chicago Tribune. https://www.chicagotribune.com/chi-neat-shape-05282014-story.html

- Comana, F. (n.d.). *Non-Exercise Activity Thermogenesis: A NEAT Approach to Weight Loss*. https://blog.nasm.org/exercise-programming/neat-approach-weight-loss

- Bodybuilding.com, & Writer, C. (2021, July 27). *BMR Calculator: Learn Your Basal Metabolic Rate for Weight Loss*. Bodybuilding.com. https://www.bodybuilding.com/fun/bmr_calculator.htm

- *"Never give up on a dream just because of the time it will take to accomplish it. The time will pass anyway." —Earl Nightingale*. (n.d.). The Foundation for a Better Life. https://www.passiton.com/inspirational-quotes/6559-never-give-up-on-a-dream-just-because-of-the

111 Dumbbell Workouts

For the Shy Gym Girl

Your Strength Training Guide to Build Muscle, Burn Fat and Grow Confidence.

By Sophie Smith

"Never give up on a dream just because of the time it will take to accomplish it. The time will pass anyway.'

~Earl Nightingale.

Printed in Great Britain
by Amazon

2572452a-0c88-468e-ac6c-496100ea6cb1R01